THE UNSOUND MIND

Best Wishes

Logan

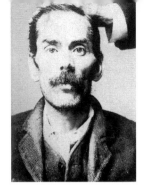

THE UNSOUND MIND

CASE HISTORIES
FROM THE CITY OF
NEWCASTLE UPON TYNE
LUNATIC ASYLUM

By

LOGAN EWING

Typeset in Dante

Editing, design, typesetting and publishing by
UK Book Publishing

www.ukbookpublishing.com

ISBN: 978-1-913179-80-9

Cover image: © Royal College of Nursing

FOR

LAURA J. EWING

AND

LISA M. EWING

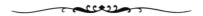

*With thanks to Ken Coates for his support,
comments and suggestions*

Contents

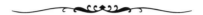

Introduction

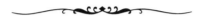

DURING 1847 IN ENGLAND and Wales, there were 5,247 patients housed in 21 County and Borough Asylums; by 1914, this had increased to 108,837 patients in 102 asylums.

When it opened in 1869, the City of Newcastle Lunatic Asylum initially accommodated 250 patients; by 1878 this number had risen to just 261. Over the coming decades, however, the city gradually, but steadily, enlarged its asylum so that by 1914, there was accommodation for almost 900 patients*.

Case histories are taken from actual case books where every entry – of varying degrees of legibility – has been made in long-hand by medical staff. The case histories highlighted relate to just a very few of the people admitted into this one asylum between the years 1869 – 1914.

**From the 1940s onwards, the number of patients accommodated at St Nicholas Hospital (previously the City of Newcastle Lunatic Asylum) fluctuated at around 1,100; as late as 1983, there was still accommodation for 850 patients – 250 admission beds and 600 long stay/elderly beds.*

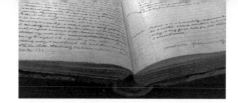

The Unsound Mind

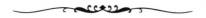

Within asylums built to last
Casebooks chronicle the unsound mind
The glimpsing of a hidden past
Untold tales are what we find

An institution, a place apart
Routine and order – a truth belied
Revealed, a world severe and stark
But who are they who reside inside?

Every walk of life is there
Each in tragedy is soaked
The unsound mind exposed, laid bare
Embattled when fear provoked

A hostage to unquiet dreams
A social outcast in all but name
A life rough-hewn, worn smooth it seems
Yet,
This is a person just the same

LOGAN EWING, 2016

Index of Case Histories

(*P = Photograph*)

MALE

FEMALE

Male Case Histories

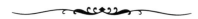

WILLIAM JAMES TAYLOR

Date of Admission: 24ᵗʰ June 1865

Background

20-year-old William, a former 'Hammerman', had previously spent a few months under the care of the Union Workhouse in the parish of St Nicholas, Newcastle. According to the Master of the Workhouse, William had been arrested and taken there as a teenager by the police after becoming violent towards his mother. William had broken 'everything in the house' and had done so several times before; his behaviour was attributed to the epileptic fits he experienced which caused him to be a danger to others whenever he 'became excited'.

Admission

It was determined by the Committee of Justices for the Borough and County of Newcastle at the time, that William should be boarded out to the Durham County Asylum at Sedgefield – chargeable to the St Nicholas Parish Union, Newcastle – and so was admitted there on 16th July 1860. During his time at Sedgefield, William was described as 'sullen and morose'; was incapable of taking care of himself and was very violent in his behaviour. Once the 'Temporary Newcastle Lunatic Asylum' in Bensham, Gateshead had opened, William was transferred there 'in a fit condition of bodily health', on 24th June 1865. Between then and his subsequent transfer at the end of 1869 to the new asylum in Gosforth, William had consistently been very noisy and violent, at times 'sauntering about using vile language'.

Violent Denunciations

William's violent behaviour remained unchanged over the next year or so and by the end of 1871 he was considered to be – in manner and appearance – 'more like a gorilla than a human being'. William required a great deal of close supervision throughout these years because of his continued 'destructive, dangerous and filthy' behaviour – and also because of the severe epileptic seizures he suffered at regular intervals. Early in 1874, William was confined to bed suffering from leg ulcers; although they were treated with linseed meal poultices they 'showed no disposition' to heal and so remained unhealthy in appearance – sometimes, they were made worse as William tended to irritate and pick at them. Even at rest in the recumbent position, William would occasionally strike out at anyone who approached him, but more often – when not being intermittently confined to bed – his 'violent denunciations' were usually directed against imaginary objects, causing him to punch walls or doors that inflicted lacerating wounds on his hands. During such episodes, it was evident William was trying to protect himself from some unseen enemy, often lifting up chairs and either smashing them against the wall or throwing them at anyone who came near. On one occasion, the intended victim retaliated by assaulting William, who was only prevented from serious injury by the prompt intervention of one of the attendants. William's condition remained much the same over the next two years – there was no change to his mental state; he was dirty in his habits and was regarded as a constant danger to himself and other people. During this period, William would invariably either be the victim of assault from other patients due to his disruptive behaviour or he would punch others 'on the nose' because they were laughing at him as he attempted to strike out at imagined opponents. After years of such behaviour, however, William was regarded as less dangerous to others as he had been in the past; by October 1877, he was now being referred to as that 'poor fellow' – someone who occasionally bruised his fists by punching walls. Nevertheless, over the following few years, William remained impulsive and unpredictable and still occupied a single room at night because he could be 'extremely noisy'.

Moody Frame of Mind

By 1881, William continued with his impulsive and reckless behaviour although his physical health remained fairly good and his mental state was still very much the same as it always had been. Over the next few years, William was generally 'untidy and dirty' in his habits and muttered a great deal to himself, giving silly and irrelevant answers to any questions put to him. Often, William would be in a listless, moody frame of mind and apt to be aggressive, frequently hitting out at those near him without provocation. Occasionally, William would still inflict injuries upon himself by knocking his fists against the walls of the airing court or even by banging his head against the walls of his bedroom. By the mid-1880s, William was thought to be 'very stupid'; when asked how old he was, he would reply he was just two years of age – on being remonstrated with about the absurdity of this, William said perhaps he may be three years old but 'certainly not more'. The late 1880s saw William frequently disposed to become aggressive, his conversation abusive and he was liable to 'paroxysms of excitement' during which he would 'assume a threatening attitude', hitting out at anyone who happened to be nearby. In April 1890, there was no change to record in William's circumstances and he continued to be 'noisy, restless, aggressive and violent', remaining so throughout the early 1890s. In 1892, for example, and in a 'paroxysm of violence', William would sometimes rush forward headlong and lash out at any person – or thing – that happened to be in his way. Such incidents flared up from time to time over the next year or so, during which William could become very quarrelsome and – quite suddenly – violent. William's state of chronic excitement had changed little over the years and on 10th April 1894 – almost twenty-five years after his initial admission – he was still noted to be 'restless, excited and violent, untidy, dirty and mischievous, incoherent and unable to converse intelligently'. Despite his debilitating mental state, William had always remained in fairly good physical health but in February 1895, he fell injuring his shoulder and whilst some bruising was evident, no fracture or dislocation had been detected. As a precaution, however, William's arm was bandaged and strapped to his side and he was confined to bed until, two weeks later, he was able to move his arm without any pain – by May he had reverted back again to being 'excited, noisy, troublesome, quarrelsome and violent'. On 4th June, William became ill and coughed up thick and purulent mucous during the night; on examination, his lungs were found to be congested and he was thought to have suffered a severe attack of 'colic with syncope'. William remained in feeble health and on bed-rest for the next few weeks but quickly regained his strength and made a good recovery from what had now been diagnosed as phthisis. By November, it was noted William was much thinner than he used to be and that his behaviour was generally quieter than usual. Throughout 1896, William slowly recovered and he gradually returned to his previous state of being 'restless, dirty and violent' – now, however, his physical health was not as good as it had been previously. By the end of that year, William's physical health declined once more as he suffered from the occasional attack of syncope which, in turn, meant he became less excitable and his assaults on the walls of buildings less frequent.

An Untidy Old Dement

William remained susceptible to violent outbursts and during restless periods would continue to fight imaginary people, state his name was 'Jimmy Taylor' and that he was two-years-old. Over the next few years, William's physical health improved slightly but mentally there was little change as he continued to hallucinate and act 'very impulsively'. On 20th January 1899, William was described as an 'untidy old dement' who scarcely conversed and often violently punched himself on the face – evidence of which, on one occasion, presented itself as an 'abrasion over the molar bone'. Such behaviour continued into the following year when William would still 'batter his face', noisily shout in response to his hallucinations and violently attack other patients whilst under the influence of his 'senile fancies'. At the beginning of February 1901, William became unwell again and suffered a 'syncopal attack' during a walk around the grounds. A few weeks later, William had partly recovered but remained 'rather feeble', suffering from what was now thought to be cardiac dyspnoea. William's condition deteriorated further in April and he was unable to eat properly or sleep very well at night because of his difficulty in breathing. By 1st May, William had become much weaker and he started refusing the small doses of digitalis prescribed for his heart condition. On the evening of 7th May, William suffered a syncopal attack and although he made a slight recovery, William fatally suffered another one at 11.30pm. At 12.15am on 8th May 1901, 60-year-old William died of heart disease, having first been admitted to asylum care as a 20-year-old man.

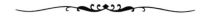

PATRICK HENRY

Date of Admission: 22nd January 1869

Background

Patrick was a 58-year-old unmarried labourer with a criminal past, who had spent some time in Portsmouth prison; he believed his brother had been murdered in the workhouse and that his assassins were now coming after him. Patrick thought these assassins were crawling around under the floor of his house and plotting the best method of how to 'annihilate' him – such was his agitation that Patrick was described as 'that poor fellow who was in constant turmoil'.

Admission

Patrick's condition was diagnosed as one of 'syphilitic insanity' as he continued to persist in the belief his brother had been murdered – even though the Medical Superintendent of the asylum had recently met his brother. Over the next few years, Patrick remained convinced of his brother's death and that his murderers were now trying to kill him; Patrick believed if he slept underneath the mattress of his bed at night, he could help avoid this happening. By 1874, the delusions relating to his brother's murder and the perceived attempts on his own life continued to greatly distress Patrick – his disquiet now so severe he was unable to do any work at all around the ward during the day and he continued to be very noisy and disruptive at night. During this period, Patrick often sought out the doctor when he arrived on his daily visit to the ward; having done so, he would rush up to him to plead his case and ask the doctor how long he was 'to be kept here to be murdered?'. The beginning of 1875 saw little improvement in Patrick's circumstances and he became increasingly troublesome, frequently running after anyone who entered the ward and confronting them with his incoherent ramblings. Nor was there any respite at night as Patrick noisily stuffed his bedsheets and blankets against the door and window of his bedroom in order to keep out the murderers he believed were out there – somewhere – looking for him.

Eccentric Manner

By February 1875, Patrick had resorted to 'plugging up' his ears and nostrils with paper so that his would-be murderers could be prevented from blowing steam into them as part of their insidious attempts to kill him. The Ward Doctor had now begun visiting Patrick every evening to try and persuade him to remove the wooden wedges that Patrick had started to insert under his bedroom door in order to prevent it being opened from the outside during the night. Even when the wedges were successfully taken away, Patrick would simply replace them with his pillows and chamber pot; such precautions were sometimes not enough for him, however, and Patrick would turn his bed completely around in the dark to barricade the door – doing so within 'a few seconds' of the doctor leaving. Towards the end of that year – despite various altercations with fellow patients – some improvement was noted in Patrick's general conduct when it came to bedtime. No wedges were now found under his door, nor were his bedding and clothes being used in 'the eccentric manner' to which they had previously been employed – such progress was achieved mainly because of the effectiveness of one of the medical staff visiting Patrick two or three times a night to reassure him and prevent it from happening. Nevertheless, there didn't appear to be the 'slightest hope' of any particular continued improvement in Patrick's mental state and he eventually reverted to turning his bed around again to block the bedroom door – and to resume 'filling his ears' with paper. Throughout 1876, Patrick seldom attempted to help out around the ward and he gradually became increasingly untidy in his personal appearance – made worse by the continued use of his 'devices for keeping out the steam'. Patrick would often shout out all day about his murderers – there were now four of them – and he was still frequently noisy during the night as he attempted to secure the door leading into his bedroom by blocking it from behind. Patrick was also becoming increasingly dangerous to those around him, particularly in the morning – his changes of mood self-evident as when excited, the skin over the entire surface of his body took on a bright red colour giving him 'a most peculiar appearance'.

Decline in Condition

On the morning of 21st March 1877, Patrick was observed to be suffering from intense dyspnoea; in a very weak state, Patrick was immediately transferred to the Infirmary Dormitory, located in the Second Ward, and placed on bed-rest. Upon examination, it was ascertained Patrick had sustained fractured ribs on his right-hand side which were then strapped with adhesive plaster; he was also suffering from bronchitis for which linseed oil and mustard were applied to his chest. 'Extras' to his diet, consisting of 4ozs of whisky and two pints of beef tea were prescribed daily for Patrick – as were 'special attendants', detailed to watch him day and night. Enquiries were made into the sudden decline in Patrick's physical health and how he came to sustain his fractured ribs; from the subsequent investigation, it emerged that Patrick, who, noisier than usual the previous night, had been assaulted by one of the other patients – described as someone 'very strong and violent' when excited' – who rose from his bed during the night to hit Patrick because he wouldn't be quiet – presumably entering Patrick's room on one of the few occasions when the door had not been barricaded from the inside. The patient making this claim had observed the incident – said to have been illuminated by gaslight coming from the attendant's room – and stated that although he saw Patrick being struck in the face, he did not see the protagonist do anything else. The conclusion was reached that, judging from the witness's personality and general disposition, it was thought 'more than probable' Patrick had been struck on the right side of the chest without the witness being able to observe it. No clear account could be elicited from Patrick because of his own delusions about would-be murderers pursuing him and about whom he always referred to anyway, whenever spoken to about anything.

Much Worse

A special night-watch was kept on Patrick over the next week; apart from a loss of appetite and sleeping a great deal, his condition began to improve and the night-watch was therefore discontinued on 27th March. The following night, however, Patrick's condition deteriorated and a 'mustard blister' was applied over the right side of his chest for twenty minutes followed by linseed meal poultices to be applied every hour. Patrick was also ordered half an ounce of castor oil and a special attendant was once more put on duty to watch over him. On the morning of 28th March, Patrick appeared much improved and fresh strapping was applied around the right side of his chest – but later in the evening, his condition suddenly declined again as his lips and face turned blue and he found it difficult to breathe. Patrick started coughing, gasping for air as he moaned and raved about the 'murderers of John Cail and a Catholic clergyman'. On the morning of 29th March, Patrick's tongue was very foul and dry; his nose and lips were blue from congestion and his laboured breathing continued unabated. Patrick was now finding it difficult – despite repeated doses of castor oil – to cough up the mucous from his lungs and he could 'hardly be persuaded' to take any beef tea. At around 2.15pm later that afternoon, Patrick suddenly became much weaker and he died at 2.25pm with the cause attributed to chronic bronchitis; emphysema and fracture of the 4th right rib.

On 30th March the following day, further enquiries were made into the 'supposed assault' that had occurred on the night of 20th March, resulting in the witness – patient Robert Hedley – making an additional statement alleging that the protagonist – now identified as patient James Alexander – had taken hold of Patrick by the shoulder and shoved him. Mr Hedley further alleged that Mr Alexander did not speak angrily to Patrick but was 'vexed' at him for not going to asleep and for keeping others awake. Mr Alexander now acknowledged having taken hold of Patrick by the shoulders and pressing down on him, but insisted he did not strike Patrick nor injure him in any way. The following month, on 2nd April 1877, a coroner's inquest was held; the verdict returned by the jury was that 64-year-old Patrick – having feared for years being murdered in his bed by unknown assailants – had died from chronic bronchitis and emphysema, exacerbated by a broken rib and that the 'said rib was broken by misadventure'.

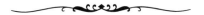

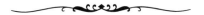

CHARLES SAVILLE

Date of Admission: 3rd March 1870

Background

Charles was a 57-year-old widower suffering from melancholia and hypochondria who believed he was dying and that all his food was turning to 'wind and water'; Charles was also convinced he had no heart, stomach and bowels because he had been badly treated in the past by a Dr Jefferson. Despite believing in the imminence of his own death, Charles nevertheless 'laboured assiduously' at a range of activities, such as showing an interest in ornithology and birds like 'larks and starlings'.

Admission

Charles persisted in the 'extraordinary delusion' he had no internal organs – or 'any insides', as he termed it, stating all his digestive organs had 'finished' about six years ago; Charles was adamant that he had never had a bowel motion since then – even though he continued to have a healthy appetite. By way of explanation, Charles declared that as soon as he eats his food, it changes into 'wind and water' and that he was able to live on the 'old blood' found inside his body from around twenty years ago. Despite such fixed beliefs, Charles proved to be a 'very useful' and trustworthy person over the next few years and was employed by staff to run errands for them – eventually, he was even given parole on a daily basis to go out beyond the asylum grounds. During this period, Charles' many delusionary beliefs remained much in evidence and he continued to assert he had no intestines or abdominal organs and that he never passed urine or defecated.

Running Errands

By March 1875, 'Old Charley' – as he was now known by staff – was well-established within the asylum and still employed in running errands on a daily basis, coping with his responsibilities 'remarkably well'. Charley also took great care of the swans and ducks, which he fed every day as they roamed around the grounds; when not working, Charley was regarded as a 'very good hand' at games such as whist and bagatelle – on occasions, he would even sing at the weekly dance, which was held every Wednesday. Charley was thought to be in very good physical health for a man of his age and he always appeared happy and contented – although inclined to be egotistical and apt to take advantage of the privileges granted to him by staff. Charley was also known to have quite an 'amiable disposition' and was observed on one occasion at the windows of one of the female wards handing out some tobacco to a female patient – a deed which resulted in him being confined to his own ward for 24 hours. Charley acknowledged the justice of this punishment and did not appear to bear anybody ill-will on account of it; not long after this incident, Charley was allowed (on parole) to attend the Newcastle Races on the 24th July where he was said to have 'behaved himself'.

Began Staying Out

Despite the relative freedom Charley enjoyed in regularly being allowed out on parole, there was no improvement in his mental state and he still 'cherished' the old delusions regarding his bodily functions. If anybody caught him in the act of performing the 'necessary operation' of going to the toilet, Charley would try and convince the observer it was down to their own imagination – indeed, he became highly indignant and considered it a personal insult they had even been looking. Nevertheless, Charley remained very trustworthy, took care of his personal appearance and was very fond of reading his Bible. Charley continued in his employment as staff messenger but he was now on a 'fixed tariff', a system of payment which depended on what he was asked to do – he could get very jealous of other patients, however, if they undertook any of these jobs for free. Charley carried on in this way without incident for the next couple of years but, towards the end of 1877, he was proving to be less trustworthy and therefore liable to be employed less often in running staff errands. It was felt that Charley could be 'rather cunning' at times in his dealings with them, as he began to take advantage of the kindness they had always shown him. Now, Charley would stay out beyond the hours agreed, sometimes coming back drunk and making 'too free' at the places he may have been sent to, as he gossiped about the affairs of the asylum. Charley would also try to overcharge for his services whenever he could and tell the 'most bare-faced lies' which, on one occasion, confined him to the ward for gross impertinence.

Charley became very anxious he should not be sent to another asylum because of his behaviour but on 24th January 1878, he was removed to the Third County Asylum of Middlesex at Banstead and 'discharged as relieved to their care'.

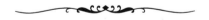

THOMAS HENRY SHAW

Date of Admission: 6th April 1871

Background

Thomas, a 36-year-old married man and a painter by trade, was suffering from a 'great depression of spirits' with occasional fits of nervous irritation and excitement – often, he would give vent to outbursts of weeping and was frequently disposed to staying in bed. It was thought Thomas had suffered a previous attack around six years ago, but it was not known whether he had received any treatment for it. Thomas says that when he was growing up, he practised masturbation and continued to do so even after he was married – attributing this, in association with drinking heavily, as being of sufficient cause for his own insanity. Thomas felt overpowered with this burden of guilt for his past life; he thought there would be no forgiveness for him and that he was about to die.

Admission

Thomas never settled during the first week of his admission and he became increasingly weak as he refused to eat; eventually, it was necessary for an attendant to feed him by spoon. Thomas was very restless and low in spirit during this period and he would often call out that he must die as the 'hand of God' was upon him. His mental state and childish manner meant Thomas often required a draught of chloral hydrate at night to help him sleep. His condition remained unchanged over the next few months, but by August, Thomas appeared 'somewhat improved' and he was a little more cheerful than he had been for some time.

Doing a Little Work

By September, Thomas was 'altogether' more cheerful, having by now written several letters to his wife – one of the attendants making the observation that Thomas could write a 'pretty fair letter'. During the day, Thomas started doing a little work around the ward such as painting various articles of furniture; in the evening, he would participate in playing cricket outside with the other patients. On the 14th October 1871, Thomas was discharged after having made his escape fourteen days beforehand.

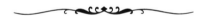

DAVID BELL

Date of Admission: 5ᵗʰ December 1872

Background

Unmarried 40-year-old David, a general labourer, had previously been a patient some years ago at lunatic asylums in County Durham and Belfast. David had been admitted to Sedgefield Asylum in County Durham again when he started writing 'incoherent letters' to a Miss Davison of Greencroft Park, the contents of which were deemed to 'prove him insane'. On 5ᵗʰ December 1872, David was transferred to the City of Newcastle Lunatic Asylum in Coxlodge.

Admission

On admission, David was restless and excited, scarcely answering any questions put to him and whilst in good physical health, he was described as being 'rather fleshy'. David had a tendency to wear a number of iron rings on the fingers of his right hand in order, he says, to counteract the effects of frostbite on his left ankle – he also wore a cotton belt around his body through which some larger iron rings were threaded; the purpose of these were not specified. Always incoherent when engaged in conversation, David was nevertheless regarded as quiet in manner even though, on occasions, he could become rather 'peevish' – an attribute thought to demonstrate an uncertain temper. Over the next two years, David continued to exhibit a 'peculiar taste in dress' and would spend a great deal of time sewing various pieces of material – and anything else he could 'get his hands on' – to his cap and clothes. David also spent the greater part of his day drawing out maps of properties he felt he owned and made various calculations in a notebook 'full of scribbling' which, he asserted, contained his own private memoranda relating to the 'concept of motion'. David often wore a large, white cloth decorated in letters and figures made from coloured wool which he draped over his shoulders as he walked around; at night, he slept with the bedclothes 'reversed' – the quilt next to his body and the bed-sheets on top of it; a gesture he made to the 'mourning memory' of his four brothers who died unmarried.

Eccentric

By June 1875, David's appearance was considered so eccentric it became 'absolutely necessary' to remove certain items that were hanging from his clothes; 7lbs 4ozs of 'old iron and rubbish' were removed – as well as the seven or eight horseshoes sewn into his cap. Also noted amongst David's possessions were: an old file; two or three knife blades and a key 'similar to that used for the shower bath'. Such eccentricity notwithstanding, David was regarded as being of a 'quiet and harmless disposition' and someone who could be industriously employed in helping out around the ward. David tended to keep himself to himself and refused to attend Chapel; he was seldom present at the weekly dances and did not participate in any of the various activities generally enjoyed by other patients. Although there was no discernible change to his mental state, David continued in good physical health and was clean in his personal habits – his propensity, however, for 'collecting rubbish' and decorating his clothes with it, remained. On the 1st November 1875, David was discharged back to Sedgefield Asylum in Durham County as not improved.

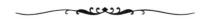

193 *Transferred from Sedgefield Asylum Max. Freudenthal aa 10th Dec 1872*

Reg. No. 639. Chronic Mania Fair. *æt. 39 years, single, clerk, Religion not known, is not the first attack, nothing is known about the previous attack nor the duration of present one – cause unknown – if epileptic unknown, is suicidal, if dangerous not known.*

MAX FREUDENTHAL

Date of Admission: 10th December 1872

Background

Max was a 39-year-old unmarried clerk who had spent two and a half years at Sedgefield Asylum, County Durham, suffering from chronic mania before he was transferred and admitted to the City of Newcastle Lunatic Asylum. In the past, Max had spent about a year and a half in an asylum somewhere in Germany after having threatened to drown himself.

Admission

On admission, Max was described as a small, excited-looking man with a 'Jewish cast of feature' who rapidly walked around, speaking quickly as he asserted his abdomen was full of drugs and his sinews 'filled with flames'. Thinking himself 'perfectly sane' – he believed he had the brain of the Emperor Napoleon and the heart of Queen Victoria – Max was convinced of his powers of persuasion and oratory, claiming to speak better than anyone in the House of Lords. Over the next twelve months, Max behaved in a very talkative and restless manner but nevertheless managed to gain employment working outside in the gardens. He was suspicious of other patients, however, and felt they couldn't be trusted because of the power he claimed they had of tapping into his senses – on one occasion, Max attacked someone with a spade for doing just this. By December 1873, Max was generally regarded as an 'extremely irritable man' who, at dinner on New Year's Eve, hit another patient – without the slightest provocation – on the face with a spoon. At first, his victim 'brooked the insult' but after a minute or two, suddenly pushed his soup bowl into his assailant's face causing two lacerations to Max's nose and right eye.

Disruptive Behaviour

Max's disruptive and excitable behaviour persisted throughout the course of 1874, thereby consolidating his reputation for being a 'very troublesome and impulsive' fellow. Upon entering 1875, Max was now chattering 'incessantly' to anyone who cared to listen to him, mainly in French but also in English and German – even demonstrating some knowledge of the Latin he had apparently acquired on the continent. Whenever the ward doctor paid a visit, Max rushed up to him and kept up a rapid, continuous conversation – the doctor, however, was often able to persuade Max to defer the conversation to a more convenient time. Over subsequent visits and after various unsuccessful attempts at conversation, Max had gradually learned not to accost the doctor who, by now, had 'ceased to notice' Max's presence. The other patients were not quite so fortunate, however, as on the 12th February, Max attacked one of them, stating he had been urged to do so by another patient; the outcome of this particular altercation was Max nearly being thrown into an open fire in retaliation. A few weeks later, on the 3rd March, Max annoyed a fellow patient twice during the weekly dance, the first time resulting in Max being kicked by this patient; towards the end of the evening, Max hit the patient again and a fight quickly ensued, but a doctor, who had been standing nearby, promptly intervened – although not before Max himself sustained a black eye and bloody nose. When asked why he had annoyed the other patient in the first place, Max replied the patient had been 'possessed of eight devils', naming several other patients whose spirits also entered him on these occasions. Max went on to state he intended to kill the ward doctor – or someone else – before very long; that he considered himself a lunatic and that nothing could be done except by placing him in a criminal asylum.

Becoming Dangerous

It was felt Max was becoming very dangerous indeed; several times now, he had attempted to kill some of the other patients and even some of the attendants – on one occasion, almost succeeding. Max was generally regarded as being at his 'most treacherous' when – unaware of his presence – he attempted to attack people from behind. Max's violent and unpredictable behaviour continued over the following weeks; in one notable incident, Max started using abusive and threatening language towards three other patients whilst they were all outside in the airing court at 10.30 in the morning. Max threw a brick at one of the men with such force, it smashed against the asylum wall; the enraged man, having just had a narrow escape, started chasing Max –who only enraged him further when Max managed to run between his legs. Having finally caught up with Max they began fighting, although each only sustained a few scratches – Max, however, also had 'some of his beard torn out'. This incident only served to reinforce the view of Max as a 'most troublesome fellow' – a view reinforced yet again the following month when Max was deprived of a large wooden nail he had sharpened and which he intended using to kill someone. Max continued to regularly exhibit abusive and aggressive behaviour, annoying others with his 'very filthy language' and sometimes attacking them without any provocation. Max was also used to being attacked himself – on two or three occasions by one particular patient who, on the 31st May, cut Max's face 'all over' – but not before Max managed to inflict an 'ugly wound' on his adversary's forehead with two pieces of iron he had managed to conceal about his person. Later that afternoon, Max managed to escape over the airing court walls only to be brought back almost immediately – but not before stating his determination to succeed in escaping 'sooner or later'. Around this time, Max had confided in medical staff his intention of running off to Stockton-on-Tees where he thought he could get a certificate of sanity from a doctor – but when asked how he would pay his expenses, Max replied he had 'tuppence to do so' and that this would be sufficient. Although still inclined to be troublesome and excitable, over the next few months, Max started to behave himself and became a little more manageable in his behaviour – although he remained very noisy and continued to use 'filthy language'. On the 1st November 1875, whilst his behaviour was still reasonable, Max was considered fit enough to travel; later that day, he was discharged and transferred back Sedgefield Asylum in County Durham as 'not improved'.

JOHN HENRY GIBSON

Date of Admission: 7th July 1874

Background

John was a 33-year-old printer and widower who, after six months of marriage, lived with his second wife, Alice, at Cromwell Street, Newcastle; for three weeks prior to his admission John had been rambling in his conversation and behaving in a strange manner. John was convinced a recent visitor to the house suspected him of wrong-doing – he also believed they had been shipwrecked together off the coast of Tynemouth three years ago.

John had recently become very emotional and changeable in his mood and was often disposed to episodes of either laughing or crying for no reason his wife could understand. The week prior to his admission, John had locked Alice out of their house then proceeded to run around wielding a large knife before standing at a window gesticulating and threatening the large crowd that had come to gather outside.

Admission

John was 'quiet and tractable' on admission, believing he had been married to his present wife for two years and that his first wife was not dead. It seemed that John's memory was 'almost totally gone' and he was unable to remember anything he said in recent conversation – when 'taxed with the utterance of some gross absurdity' John denied any recollection of having mentioned it. In the days following his admission, John started to show a 'degree of grandeur' in his bearing and would often rush up to staff in the airing court to ascertain their opinion on 'how they thought he was looking today'. After some weeks, it was noted John seemed to have 'very imperfect' control over the movement of his limbs when, on the morning of 2nd August, he suddenly fell to the floor whilst making his bed. The attendant who discovered John quickly examined him and reported that John appeared to be paralysed down the left-hand side, a complete absence of motion in his left arm was noted and only limited movement of the left leg was observed – even his slightly-protruding tongue was drooping to the left. Presumed to have suffered a stroke, John was confined to bed and prescribed bromide of potassium three times a day, supplemented by an occasional draught of castor oil when required. Over the next week or so, some movement gradually returned to John's arm and leg. With no further improvement evident over the coming months, however, John tended to spend all day sitting in an armchair and was only able to walk with assistance.

Working Outside

Continuing with the bromide of potassium treatment, by the end of the year, John was slowly showing some signs of improvement although he continued to have very little power in his left arm and was only able to move his index finger slightly. By February 1875, John's memory was regarded as 'extremely feeble' and whilst he remembered being married to Alice, he could recall little else. Despite having been admitted eight months previously, John believed it had only been a few days – 'a week ago at most' – and although now regarded as hemiplegic, he did not see himself as lame – only that he felt some numbness in his left arm and leg. Nevertheless, John's condition slightly improved over the next two years as his memory got a little better and he gradually grew stronger in his physical health; his medication was now discontinued and he became increasingly more active, regularly attending church and even singing in the choir. John also joined in various other 'amusements' and maintained a steady progress in his physical health during this period – so much so, that by the beginning of 1877, he was working outside in the grounds, showing himself to be 'very willing' in his attitude towards his duties. On the night of 11th April, however, there had been a fall of snow and whilst out working the following morning, the big toe on John's right foot was noted to be in a 'gangrenous state'. The toe was quickly treated with tincture of potassium chloride, cotton wool was applied around the toe and secured with a bandage and John was sent to bed with 'a pint of beef tea and a pint of porter (extra) per diem' ordered to aid his recovery. The foot healed well over the next two weeks and by the 24th April, the 'extras' having been discontinued, John was now up and out of bed. By the end of 1877, John's general physical health had improved further – although the paralysis of his left arm and leg was now thought to be more 'pronounced' than it had been before.

Cheerful and Obliging

Over the next few years, John's circumstances changed little, there was no change noted to his mental state and his memory remained 'very defective'.

However, John continued to sing in the choir and he was still working outside in the grounds – even regaining the use of his left arm sufficiently enough to allow him to push a wheelbarrow. Unfortunately, after suffering an attack of impetigo in 1880 which incapacitated him, John was unable to continue working outside and he was subsequently put to work helping out on the ward instead. By 1883, John's hemiplegic condition was now deemed 'less observable', and although occasionally confined to bed with arthritis, he was nevertheless described as being of a 'cheerful and obliging' disposition. Over the next few years, John's memory continued to be extremely impaired and he was unable to remember even recent events, having great difficulty in recollecting the conversation with friends who had visited only a few days previously. Nevertheless, John continued to enjoy singing in the choir and, despite his limitations, was able to perform his work duties 'regularly and efficiently'.

'Epileptiform Fits'

By April 1889, John was once more working outside in the grounds and tending to the gardens – now, however, he was 'very silly' in his general demeanour and often laughed 'immoderately' at ordinary expressions as if they were 'rich jokes'. Despite his poor memory and silly behaviour, and as well as his inability to hold a detailed conversation, John remained employed in the asylum grounds and continued to be an active member of the chapel choir – even singing occasionally at the weekly dance. As well as his hemiplegia, by April 1892, John was now thought to be labouring under partial dementia due to an underlying diagnosis of syphilis which left him 'aggressively excited' at times. John remained in good general health, however, and continued to work in the gardens; generally, he was regarded as 'quiet and civil' – with occasional episodes of excitable and abusive behaviour.

On the morning of 18th November 1893, John had three slight 'epileptiform fits' in quick succession and cried out as he fell to the floor, convulsing slightly before coming round again – then immediately going through the same process twice more in quick succession. Afterwards, John was confined to bed where he eventually recovered – four days later, however, John had three more fits in quick succession – exactly as previously experienced. Having eventually recovered, John gradually regained his health and suffered no further fits; by March 1894, he was working hard outside again and regarded as being 'quiet, cheerful and civil' in his general disposition. John continued without much change over the next few years and apart from a few epileptic seizures in 1897, he coped well with his hemiplegia and remained pleasant and contented in manner. 1900 saw a lapse in John's behaviour as he became increasingly childish and rambled in his conversation but apart from this, John ate and slept well during the following years and he remained in good enough physical health to continue working outside in the grounds. By 1907, however, John was becoming increasingly indifferent to his circumstances and took no interest in his surroundings; he was also suffering from an inguinal hernia which, after 'considerable difficulty', was reduced in October with the aid of an anaesthetic. This procedure took its toll on 66-year-old John and he spent a great deal of time recuperating in bed on the Infirmary Ward; John wasn't troubled any further by his hernia after this but he never really made a full recovery. John continued in poor physical health and over the following months, he remained in bed and only got up for part of the day. On the morning of the 6th April 1908, John was found to be in a 'very stupid and confused' state; his speech was slurred and indistinct and he had difficulty in swallowing. Despite taking a fair amount of nourishment and stimulants, John became increasingly weak as his condition deteriorated; at 07.40 on the morning of 9th April, John died; the cause attributed to lobar pneumonia and cerebral disease with hemiplegia.

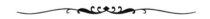

ROBERT LITTLEWOOD

Date of Admission: 19ᵗʰ October 1874

Background

Robert, aged 'about' 36 years, was a widower and a gardener by occupation; he lived in Byker, Newcastle although his next of kin – his father, William – lived in Great Yarmouth. For some weeks prior to his admission, Robert was noted to have been behaving strangely as he became increasingly excited and depressed by turns; Robert's actions were apparently influenced by the voices he heard and the visions he saw before him. This was Robert's second 'attack', the first having occurred around five years ago when he underwent treatment at Thorpe Lunatic Asylum in Norfolk.

Admission

On admission, Robert was found to be in fair physical health although he suffered from ulcers on his left foot and leg; this left him initially confined to bed whilst they were treated with linseed poultices. Mentally, Robert had a very exalted idea of his own sense of power and knowledge, considering himself to know more than any other person and that he was on a 'special mission' to speak to mankind. In asserting such beliefs, Robert was deemed to 'entertain very peculiar' religious views, in which he described a vision of heaven he claimed to have experienced when observing people being saved as they stood by a 'gaping wide and red-hot hole' leading down into hell. By the end of November, Robert was allowed out of bed every day despite occasional displays of excitable conversation, which, in the early hours of one morning, led to him attempting to violently assault another patient. A consequence of this behaviour led to Robert being removed to a single room and put into seclusion for a short period until he calmed down – further episodes of 'violent excitement' were usually followed by similar periods of seclusion.

'A Very Quarrelsome, Sullen and Impertinent Fellow'

By the beginning of 1875, Robert remained unpredictable in his behaviour; physically, he was looking 'remarkably strong and well' although his leg tended to swell up frequently, requiring him to stay in bed for a few days at a time. On the morning of 1st April – in a fit of excitement – Robert kicked in the panel of a door, doing considerable damage to its framework in the process. As well as exhibiting such behaviour, Robert was also regarded as a 'very quarrelsome, sullen and impertinent fellow' who was not inclined to undertake work of any kind. On 25th April at 3.40pm, Robert managed to escape from the asylum by climbing over the wall of an airing court – his freedom didn't last very long as he was soon discovered in a nearby house where he had lain in wait to see if he was being pursued. The attendants sent to collect him had trouble in bringing him back, however, as a mob had since gathered and was being led by a 'respectably-clad' man who acted as spokesman, inciting them to prevent Robert from being taken away – unsuccessfully, as Robert was quickly returned to the asylum where he arrived back safely just after 4.10pm.

The following day, Robert became very troublesome when outside in the airing court – this time assaulting attendants and refusing to 'return into the House' with the other patients. Eventually – persuasion being ineffective – Robert had to be carried inside by four attendants and 'removed' to a more secure ward where he stayed until the 10th May when he returned to his own ward after having gradually settled down. Two weeks later, however, Robert's troublesome behaviour meant he was back on the Second Ward – his behaviour now included goading other patients to misbehave and trying to dissuade them from going to work. Robert continued to assault any patient he felt was annoying him – matters took a more serious turn on the 3rd July, when Robert came across a half-brick in the airing court and took the opportunity to throw it through the Assistant Medical Officer's sitting-room window. This was done with such force that as well as taking pieces of the window frame out, it also damaged the door on the opposite side of the room. If the Assistant Medical Officer had been sitting at his desk – which he had vacated only a few minutes earlier – he would 'almost certainly' have been killed.

Violent

On 4th July, Robert was able to break the lock of his bedroom door but was quickly restrained and prevented from inflicting further damage to it; when his clothes were searched, a very sharp piece of serrated steel 'shaped like a knife blade' was found in his pockets – as well as a large nail that had apparently been recently sharpened. Only two days later, at 4.30pm on 6th July, Robert shattered the door of another single room in which he had been placed. This resulted in the removal of his bedstead as it was considered 'very probable' he had used it as a battering ram to attack the door. At 8pm that evening, Robert received a draught of chloral hydrate sedative which appeared to have no discernible effect on him as, only half an hour later, he proceeded to smash the window shutter of yet another single room to which he had subsequently been moved. The Medical Officer therefore felt he had no choice but to now place Robert in a canvas strait-jacket – but he was so violent, it required the efforts of the Head Attendant and four attendants to get him into it. The following morning, Robert appeared to have regretted his recent behaviour and was 'very penitent' with regards to it, acknowledging that staff had acted correctly in restraining him. The strait-jacket was therefore removed, and Robert was allowed to mix with the other patients; he conducted himself well for the rest of the day – but as a precaution, he still received another draught of chloral hydrate at bedtime that night. This improvement in his behaviour did not appear to last very long as, on 28th July, Robert destroyed the clothes he was wearing, requiring him to be dressed with 'canvas clothing' and an attendant assigned to keep him under close supervision. That night, Robert's bedstead was again removed from his room and he was provided with 'strong rugs' to sleep under instead – but he still managed to destroy them (and the shirt he was wearing). The next day, Robert promised he would behave better in future – a promise that lasted all of two days as on 31st July, Robert made a 'partial escape' by once more climbing over the wall of an airing court before concealing himself on a hillock near the laundry; he was quickly brought back after an absence of about ten minutes.

A Danger to Others

Despite being described as otherwise 'clean in his habits' and generally careful with his personal appearance, Robert continued to be 'very troublesome' in his behaviour. Throughout August and September, he was still fighting with other patients and annoying staff at every opportunity – for example, throwing stones from the airing court up at the windows of attendants' bedrooms. On one such occasion, Robert broke three panes of glass which resulted in him being placed under the charge of two attendants – no easy task for the staff as he would invariably throw himself to the ground and try to kick and injure them whenever they attempted to get him to stand back up. Robert's disruptiveness continued into October; often blackening the eyes of both staff and patients in the various fights he seemed to get embroiled in. After one incident, attempts were made to restrict Robert's movements by placing him into a 'camisole' but when three members of staff tried to do so, he 'struck and kicked right and left' before finally being overpowered and restrained. After eventually settling down, Robert promised to behave himself – as he usually did – but even so, he was still regarded as a danger to others – indeed, he was deemed to be 'about the worst disposed patient in the House'. Not only was Robert destructive and annoying to those around him, he would often instigate trouble between one patient and another, endeavouring to cause unrest and dissatisfaction amongst everyone else. Because of this, Robert wasn't allowed to undertake any work around the ward or even outside in the gardens but as the months passed, his behaviour and general conduct slowly began to improve again. Now, he was sometimes permitted to attend 'Divine Service' and be present at various social functions – the only untoward incident occurring on 14th December when he was disarmed of a large knife he had fashioned out of an old piece of metal. By January 1876 – and for the following few months – Robert's behaviour deteriorated once more as he became increasingly excited and abusive, stating his intention and determination to 'break out of the asylum'. Robert also seemed determined to persist in his aggressive behaviour, as highlighted on 28th February when he broke another patient's nose in an unprovoked attack; soon after, part of an old knife he had been observed sharpening was found in one of his pockets. Robert's troublesome nature slowly subsided – despite the occasional fight with other patients – and in March, he started helping out around the ward – reluctantly it appears, claiming it went 'greatly against the grain' for him to do so.

Transferred

At the end of July, Robert was transferred to the Infirmary Ward suffering from an inflammation of the knee joint – a condition that did not prevent him from being noisy at night and abusive to other patients. After treatment, the inflammation subsided and by the end of August, Robert was transferred to the Second Ward; on 16th September and after a period of stability in his mental state, Robert was transferred back to the First Ward. Two days later, he commenced working in the grounds with a garden party, an occupation that continued until Robert was discharged recovered, on 22nd December 1876.

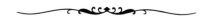

> 369
>
> *Reg No 741* Peter Gallagher ad 8th November 1874
>
> Male at 34, single, from a labourer, Roman Catholic, this his first attack has lasted one week & came on when he was 34 years of age, its cause is not known & he has not been under previous treatment; He is not known to be subject to Epilepsy, he is not suicidal but is dangerous to others.

PETER GALLAGHER

Date of Admission: 8th November 1874

Background

Peter was a 34-year-old single man who worked as a labourer and had never previously been treated; his first episode of being mentally unwell had now lasted for one week. According to Peter's sister, Hannah Bearney, with whom he lived, Peter had set fire to the house and had attempted to take the life of her husband with a hammer. Consequently, she felt that Peter was 'dangerous and beyond control'.

Admission

Over the next week or so, Peter appeared to be in a 'state of sub-acute excitement' although this had largely been alleviated by his confinement to bed. On occasions, he would refuse his meals – but never for more than a 'meal or two' at a time. When Peter was asked any questions, his usual reply was 'God knows – I don't'. Eleven days after his admission, Peter was allowed up; by 7th December, he was working regularly outside in the gardens. On Christmas Day 1874, Peter was discharged home as recovered.

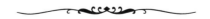

THOMAS BRUCE

Date of Admission: 29th December 1874

Background

Thomas was a 19-year-old labourer who lived with his father at Wellington Terrace, Newcastle upon Tyne. For the previous six weeks, Thomas had believed three people were trying to poison him and that there were 'openings into his head' from which animals emerged and ran down the side of his body. Regarded as being 'bent on self-destruction', Thomas was deemed to be a danger to others, having recently brandished a poker and a knife as if to strike out at those around him. According to his father, Thomas would sit quietly by the fireside, breaking his silence only to talk about the people he felt were trying to poison him.

Admission

With his heart rate 'excited and throbbing' upon admission, Thomas rambled in his conversation and complained of a 'cracking pain' in the frontal region of his head; he gradually settled over the next few weeks but remained 'moody and dull' in manner. During this initial period, Thomas appeared indifferent to his surroundings and wore a 'vacant and cheerless' facial expression as he ruminated on some perceived impending calamity. Despite such preoccupations, over the next month or so Thomas sometimes agreed, when asked, to help out around the ward and began to spend time 'loitering about the grounds' assisting the gardener in his duties – it was felt, however, that Thomas tended, as a rule, not to 'fatigue himself' by undertaking any particularly hard work. In February 1875, his general behaviour deteriorated and he started hitting out at other patients for no apparent reason.

Escape

On the morning of 17th June, Thomas escaped from a working party only to be brought back the following day by police who found him a few miles away 'acting in a disorderly manner' in Leazes Park, in the centre of Newcastle. On his return, it was noted Thomas had a scratch on his left hand as a result of being handcuffed by police after violently attempting to break out of the taxi cab returning him to the asylum. On arrival, Thomas immediately had a warm bath and was examined by a doctor who found no 'marks of violence' upon his person – other than the scratch caused by the handcuffs. A few weeks later, on the 9th July, Thomas became excitable after dinner, stating the food he had just eaten was poisoned; his behaviour remained volatile and on 25th July, he assaulted another patient by punching him and giving him a black eye. Thomas' disturbed behaviour continued as he then proceeded to tear at, and destroy, his own clothing and bedding – actions that necessitated him having to be dressed in a 'canvas suit' and placed in 'strong rugs' at bedtime that night to prevent him causing any further damage or injury to himself. Over the next few weeks, Thomas was subjected to sudden attacks of an 'acute and dangerous kind' – highlighted by being forcibly removed from two of the 'Wednesday Dances' because of his disruptive behaviour. On 5th September Thomas again became very violent and destructive, necessitating his removal to the Second Ward and only allowed to return to the First Ward a fortnight later when his behaviour improved. Having returned, Thomas promptly became involved in an argument with another patient and proceeded to knock out some of his front teeth. Apart from such incidents, Thomas was nevertheless generally clean in his habits, tidy in his personal appearance and – his past record of aggressive behaviour notwithstanding – was sometimes still allowed to attend Chapel and the weekly dance. On occasions, Thomas would assist in cleaning the ward for the sake of some 'little extra indulgences' made available to him, but otherwise, Thomas was regarded as someone who was 'lazy, excitable and dangerous to others'.

More Escapes

In February 1876, Thomas was in good physical health, had been well-behaved for some time and was assisting the attendants usefully around the ward. This good behaviour was only to last a few months, however, as on the evening of 17th June, Thomas became violently excited and attacked another patient, swearing that he was determined to kill him. It was proving difficult to keep both of them apart so Thomas was placed in seclusion for an hour and given a draught of chloral hydrate to help settle him – an approach that had the desired effect as Thomas' aggression subsided for the next two weeks or so. His aggression may have subsided, but his desire to leave the asylum remained and saw Thomas involved in a series of attempted escapes, commencing on 5th July when he succeeded in running away from a working party – only to be brought back by a policeman the following evening. This incident was soon followed by a number of other attempts during August, which usually resulted in Thomas being returned to the asylum a few hours later – some attempts only lasting about five or ten minutes. On one such occasion, Thomas escaped into the asylum grounds at 11.15am; at 11.25am he was found concealed in the stables where he violently resisted being brought back to the ward. The frequency of further attempts to escape then dwindled for a few months, but the following year Thomas renewed his efforts and on 20th March 1877 he made a particular attempt to escape by picking the bathroom door-lock on the ward with a piece of old iron. Having done so, he removed the check-blocks from one of the windows which prevented it from opening fully in order to climb through and effect his escape. When he was inevitably caught, Thomas was given a shower bath for one and a half minutes and once more removed to the Second Ward. Other attempts followed in April, including one when he tried to pick an airing court door with a 'stout wire' he had secretly acquired and managed to fashion into a pick-lock. A week after this, and in the company of another patient, Thomas and his accomplice went to the toilet, removed the seat from a toilet-bowl and descended into the sewage – but they were soon missed and quickly caught before they could make good their escape. In yet another incident on 26th May, Thomas took advantage of the temporary absence of several attendants from the ward (who all had to be present at an inquest in Newcastle) and escaped at 3.25pm into the grounds of the asylum. Five minutes later, Thomas was discovered hiding in the stable loft by a farm servant and brought back to the ward – but not before Thomas had tried to push the servant from the ladder leading up to the loft.

Slovenly and Lazy

Over the next few years Thomas's mental state gradually deteriorated and whilst he remained 'very silly' and dangerous to others, he did not exhibit the same tendency to escape that had been so prevalent before. Thomas was now less disposed to be quarrelsome but nevertheless, he refused to engage in any form of occupation; over time, however, Thomas eventually agreed to join in some of the ward's household duties and to work in the grounds again. During the early half of the 1880s, Thomas was still inclined to be of 'slovenly untidy habits' and apt to be lazy when not supervised, but otherwise, some improvement in his mental state was noted – especially with regards to his 'powers of attention'. The second half of the decade again saw a gradual deterioration in Thomas's mental state as he started to constantly mutter to himself, claiming to be twelve years of age and that he had been alive fifty years ago – Thomas also believed that he had died three times. Despite such a decline in his mental state, Thomas was still able to work outside as part of a gardening squad, but he now required a great deal of supervision in order for him to do so.

Thin and Emaciated

Mentally, his condition remained unchanged and by 1890, Thomas was being described as 'taciturn and reserved' and impossible to engage in a rational conversation. In January of that year, Thomas suffered from psoriasis to the chest and abdomen which promptly responded to a 'soda hydrosulphur' lotion and daily baths. Otherwise, Thomas's circumstances changed little during this decade – his mental state remained much the same; he was solitary; slovenly in his habits and talked in an incoherent manner. Thomas continued to exhibit many of his old delusions during this period, occasionally becoming restless and excited as he insisted he was only twenty-one years old. Despite such problems, Thomas remained in good physical health and continued to work outdoors under supervision. As the 1890s progressed, Thomas seldom spoke and was deemed to be 'labouring under chronic mania' as he continued to suffer from periods of restless excitement. Upon entering 1900, Thomas was still in fair bodily health and his mental state remained unchanged – evidence of which was his constant assertion he was only twenty-one-years old. Over the next few years his chronic mania meant Thomas could at times be quarrelsome, irritable and incoherent, whilst at others, he was largely indifferent to his circumstances. During these years, Thomas was described as 'unchangeable in every way' but despite such chronic mental health problems, Thomas had always enjoyed good physical health and continued working outdoors. In July 1908, however, his physical health began to decline and Thomas was found to be suffering from heart disease which sometimes confined him to bed; in every other respect Thomas remained the same. At the end of February 1910, Thomas was sent to bed suffering from pneumonia which, over the next few months, didn't seem to be clearing up. In April, therefore, Thomas was sent over to the nearby isolation hospital, located within the grounds of the asylum, to be cared for there. Thomas showed no signs of improvement at all over the next two months; by 1st July, he was becoming very feeble, emaciated and thought to be 'rapidly going downhill'. On 4th July 1910, after his condition had continued to deteriorate, fifty-four-years-old Thomas died at 10am of pulmonary tuberculosis, having spent the last thirty-five years of his life as a patient in the asylum.

> 509
> *Reg No*
> 801.
>
> William, Skeldon. Hodgson admitted 6th Jan'y 1876
> Male – 25 years of age – single – Poor – a boot-rivetter – Church
> of England – Previous place of abode, 44 Mill Lane, Bentick
> Newcastle-on-Tyne – Not the first attack – 24 years of age
> on first attack – Never under care & treatment – Duration
> of existing attack, one day – Supposed cause is
> unknown – Is not subject to Epilepsy, but is Suicidal
> and dangerous to others – Chargeable to the Common
> Fund of the Newcastle-on-Tyne Poor Law Union.

WILLIAM SKELDON HODGSON

Date of Admission: 6th January 1876

Background

William was a 25-year-old unmarried boot-riveter who had difficulty sleeping as he often heard noises throughout the night. At times, he would suddenly become 'taciturn' in manner for no apparent reason; according to his mother, William had threatened to cut her throat on many occasions – on the morning of his admission he had actually attempted to carry this out. Afterwards, William was discovered hiding in his bed having cut off his left testicle and mutilating the right one – he explained they were offensive to him and it was his duty to remove them.

Admission

When admitted, 'sallow-faced' William – described as 'above average height with a well-developed muscular system' – was quiet in his general disposition although his 'eye had a suspicious look'. William was allocated a single room in the Infirmary on the Third Ward, with an attendant detailed to keep him under constant observation. William's injuries were then carefully examined and treated. The wounds – having been temporarily dressed – were still haemorrhaging heavily, leaving him very weak from loss of blood. Once the dressings were removed, the left side of William's scrotum – amid a mass of coagulated blood and vascular tissue – was seen to be mutilated, leaving the remains of what were thought to be his left testicle. During careful cleansing of the wound, a sudden jet of bright red blood sprang from the coagulated mass; in searching for the cause of the bleeding, the mass subsequently became detached and was promptly removed. The jet of blood was quickly stemmed but, nevertheless, considerable arterial oozing continued for quite some time before bleeding was 'nearly entirely' overcome by elevating the scrotum. Lint, steeped in lotion, was then carefully applied over the wound with compresses placed on either side and supported by a 'T-bandage'. Upon further examination of the groin area, an irregular wound was revealed on the upper right-hand side of the scrotum, laying bare the exposed testicle. The penis itself, however, had been left undamaged. William 'trembled' throughout this procedure and his skin was moist and clammy but he did not complain of any pain except for when the wound was actually being treated. After the wound had been dressed, William appeared faint and weak but seemed to revive after being given a 'small quantity of brandy and water'. William was then able to answer questions rationally, stating he had mutilated himself with a table knife but owing to its bluntness had to make four or five cuts before eventually 'effecting his purpose'. Evidently not being 'wholly successful' in his endeavours, William now asked the doctor treating him to remove the other testicle – even stating he 'considered it proper' the penis itself should also be removed.

Alleviating Discomfort

After being made to wear a camisole to restrict his movements, William was kept in bed with a pillow positioned under the perineum and a 'hot jar' placed under his feet to keep him warm. The bed, previously prepared with four pieces of wood projecting from it (two on each side), had two sheets attached to them to cover and bind William's legs and prevent him from disturbing the dressings; a 'cradle' was placed over the pelvis to keep the weight of the bed-clothes off his body. Such measures appeared to alleviate William's general discomfort, although he complained the camisole he was wearing was 'cramping' him. William had had nothing to eat or drink all day and so was given some 'cold tea and beef tea and custard' which he appeared to enjoy very much; afterwards, William asked if he could have a cigarette – a request that was refused. Throughout the day, William was frequently seen by the Medical Superintendent and various other doctors in order to monitor his progress and to ensure his condition remained stable. Later that evening, William was given a draught of morphine to settle him down but he was reported to have vomited it up and, as a result, spent a restless and sleepless night. In the morning, William appeared to have made a slight improvement; he remained quite taciturn, however, stating to his doctor that something had told him to 'do what he had done' – adding he had recently been playing with some lads and one of them had struck him with a knee to the groin. According to William, his left testicle had never been right since, but even before this episode had occurred, William was afraid he was suffering from syphilis – his father confirming to the doctor that William had, in fact, previously been receiving treatment for this disease. Later that afternoon, William informed the Medical Superintendent he 'fancied he could see friends' in his room although he knew them to be far away; he also complained of noises in his ears and of voices telling him something. Later that morning, William's injuries were re-dressed and he was thought to have a 'very healthy appearance'. Afterwards, his camisole having been removed for a little while, William was able to sit up in bed and read a book. In the evening, once he had received some 'beef tea and an ordinary diet', William was given a draught of chloral hydrate to help him sleep that night – he initially refused to accept it before being told that if he didn't take it he would be 'compelled' to do so. On the morning of 9th January – only two days after his admission – an improvement was already being noted in his physical condition as his injuries started to heal. Later in the day, William's father contacted staff and informed them his son had always been 'a sober, steady working man' before adding that, some time ago, William had previously been under medical treatment and had requested the removal of his left testicle – a request the doctor at the time refused to agree to. William's father also said his son had recently taken to drinking his own urine every day, studying his Bible 'very intently' and engaging various clergymen in conversation – conversations which seemed to have had a profound effect on him.

'Perplexed in Mind and Body'

William's physical condition was said to be 'progressing favourably' over the next few days; he was sleeping better, his appetite had improved and he now seemed 'quite cheerful'. By 22nd January, the surface of the wound to William's scrotum was granulating well with the 'lotion and plaster dressing' now replaced by a bread poultice. A few days later, the bread poultice was removed and zinc ointment applied as the wound slowly healed. William's mental condition, however, was still a cause for concern as he stated he felt 'perplexed in mind and body' and that he had been having conversations with imaginary people. In referring to his recent actions, William declared he had a 'sudden impulse' to injure himself – before adding he had no intention of doing anything like that ever again. William's movements remained restricted as he continued to wear the camisole although, on two occasions, its sleeves were discovered untied without the attendant being aware of it. On the evening of 28th January, William was found out of bed and standing restlessly by the door of the Infirmary Dormitory at 2.15am; after this, an attendant was placed by his bed to 'monitor his every movement' at night. William was allowed to mix with other patients during the day but on one occasion, whilst freed from restraint in order to allow him some exercise, William – by some kind of 'stratagem' – induced one of the attendants to go and fetch him an orange. William then took this opportunity to 'spring through a window-sash' before any of the other attendants could intercept him – one, however, just managed to seize William before he could 'extricate himself totally' from the window. Over the next few days William was described as having a 'suspicious look about his eyes'.

By 8th February, William was expressing suicidal thoughts which compelled him to ask one of the attendants to cut his throat. Despite such behaviour,

William was allowed to have the polka (an alternative to the camisole) he was wearing to restrict his movements removed for an hour at a time – to be increased by an hour each day if he remained settled. This approach met with some success as by 16th February, William seemed much better 'in every respect' with the polka now being removed for up to six hours at a time. On 20th February, William was released from the polka for around thirteen hours and by the following day, it was discontinued altogether. William's wound had now healed up completely and by the end of the month, he was being allowed to exercise in the airing court and to assist the attendants in their duties – specifically requesting to be allowed to work outside in the grounds.

Felt Troubled

The improvements to William's bodily health and in his mental condition were maintained throughout March and April though an attempt had been made to escape from a walking party on 7th May. Despite this episode, the general improvement in William's condition was sustained over the next two months – so much so, that on 28th July, William was 'liberated on trial' until 20th December. On 27th September, however, William returned to the asylum stating he felt worse and did not feel comfortable at home. Despite being treated well by his family, William had wanted to come back as he felt troubled by his inability to find work. William was therefore placed in the Second Ward under special supervision and given a physical examination which found no abnormalities – although it was noted the left testicle was absent from his scrotum. Eating and sleeping well, William appeared to settle back into life in the asylum straight away despite occasionally appearing a bit restless and suspicious. At the beginning of October, William was transferred to the First Ward and started working in the grounds again before being moved on to assist the asylum engineer as a stoker. At 1.30pm on 14th November, William managed to escape whilst the engineer was on his dinner-break. Since no information had been received concerning his whereabouts in the meantime, William was discharged as 'recovered (after escape)' on 28th November 1876.

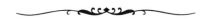

HENRY SCOTT HOOD

Date of Admission: 13th August 1877

Background

Henry was a 26-year-old single man with no known occupation, who lived at home with his parents. His father, John, stated: 'my son has suffered from epilepsy for the last fifteen years and last night, he escaped from my custody and rushed out into the street partially-clothed, he behaved so violently he was arrested by the Police who detained him in custody with my consent. I am unable to control him'.

Admission

Henry was referred to as a person of a 'low order' of intelligence with the 'aspect of a confirmed imbecile'; he was also subject to attacks of epilepsy which had never previously been treated. Described as having a low, projecting forehead and a head – small and narrow – that was cast downwards, Henry tended to 'slaver at the mouth' and breathe mainly through his nostrils. Soon after he was admitted, Henry fell into an apparent epileptic coma and made a continuous humming sound when attempts were made to rouse him. Eventually coming round, Henry uttered a complaint of pain when his chest was examined, was unable to reply to questions and was incapable of protruding his tongue when requested. On further examination, the pupils of Henry's eyes – especially the right pupil – were dilated; there was acne on his back and there were bruises and abrasions all over his body and legs. Henry was assigned to the Third Ward in the 'Second Epileptic Dormitory' with a night attendant instructed to visit him every hour. The following day, Henry seemed more coherent in his speech, although he remained 'stupid and stubborn' in appearance.

Confined to Bed

Henry was generally regarded as 'quite demented' and someone who regularly suffered from epileptic seizures. At times he was 'violently and viciously' resistive to treatment and would refuse to take his medication. In between seizures Henry was apt to be 'rather more excited than formerly' and was therefore unable to properly occupy himself. His seizures increased in frequency and severity over the next few years, which often resulted in Henry being confined to bed for 'many days at a time'. At 4.20am on the morning of 11th August, 1880, the night attendant found Henry dead, lying on the floor beside his bed; his body was resting partially on his knees and his chin was supported by the night stool. Henry's lips and nostrils were free and the expression on his face was placid. The apparent cause of his death was epilepsy.

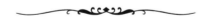

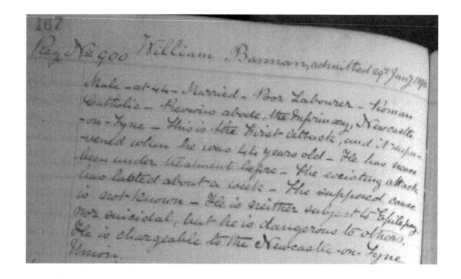

WILLIAM BANNAN

Date of Admission: 29th January 1878

Background

William was a 44-year-old married labourer whose address was listed as the 'Infirmary', Newcastle; the address of his wife, Elizabeth, was given as North Shields Workhouse. For about a week before his admission, William had been talking incoherently, stating he hadn't been receiving his proper medicine at the Infirmary; instead, he had been given some 'red stuff' which he believed was intended to poison him. According to a nurse at the Infirmary, William had accused everyone there of conspiring against him, adding that William had severely bitten the finger of one of the medical staff whilst trying to attack him with a knife.

Admission

On admission, William was assigned to the First Ward and placed in a single room where sulphur ointment was rubbed over the areas of his body affected by the itching from which he claimed to be suffering. On examination, William appeared to have little control over his limbs because of a 'want of co-ordination' in the muscles of his arms and legs; one tooth was missing from the left side of his lower jaw and several other teeth appeared to be damaged. The poor state of William's general physical condition was compounded by a severe bruise noted on his left arm, said to be the result of a blow from a poker inflicted by a porter at the Infirmary. William also claimed to have suffered from gonorrhoea in the past, although no evidence of this could be ascertained – he was, however, covered in scabies and the remains of what appeared to be a syphilitic rash, both thought to be the probable causes of his itching. William did not sleep very well over the first few nights and on one occasion was incontinent of urine and faeces. William complained of feeling very sick but when prompted to be more specific about the symptoms, he replied with a threatening look – 'oh, you know well enough what you have done to me'.

By the following week and having been nursed in bed, his scabies had almost disappeared, and William was now able to walk with some assistance and to sit up in a chair for most of the day. By the end of February, William was walking around the ward unaided, but concern still remained over his mental state. In one incident, he fell to his knees and begged forgiveness from a visiting doctor for any bad language or injuries he might have inflicted upon him when he was 'out of his mind'. As he did so, William handed the doctor a 'very insane' letter in which he implored the doctor not to kill him but to spare his life 'for the sake of his unfortunate wife and family'. At various other times, William would become very excitable and start shouting 'three cheers for the red, white and blue' whenever he was approached by someone. William was seemingly unable to fully control his limbs and appeared to be suffering from 'chorea', a condition for which he was unwilling to accept any medicine – 'shower baths' were therefore prescribed as an alternative method of treatment. William was subsequently given regular shower baths – of one-minute duration – every other morning, their beneficial effects being thought to help him gradually become a little stronger. Even so, the movements of his limbs were deemed to be 'not as regular' as they had been before.

Violent Behaviour

One day – as every male patient was having tea in the Dining Hall – William managed to conceal himself in the surgery opposite the doctor's office. The doctor, on hearing William walk about, came out of his office and went over to the surgery, offering to take him back onto the ward. When the doctor strode over to the door to lead him out, William, who was on the doctor's right side and a little behind him, 'suddenly and without any warning', punched the doctor violently in the right eye with his clenched fist and managed to trip him up. When the doctor fell to the ground, William 'sprang upon him' and bit his nose and cheek, tore at his mouth with one hand and attempted to strangle him with the other. William had almost succeeded in strangling the doctor when the noise of somebody nearby caused him to relax his hold for a second, allowing the doctor to hurriedly escape into his office and lock the door.

Very soon after this incident, William was being helped by an attendant to get undressed at bedtime when he managed to strike the attendant a violent blow, cutting and blackening his eye. This resulted in William being given a strong sedative and put into seclusion for nine hours. Despite feeling nauseous and refusing to eat at the end of this period, William was kept there for a further nine hours to ensure he had settled down sufficiently; having done so, William was then 'comparatively quiet' and managed to sustain his good behaviour for the next couple of weeks.

Eventually, William was able to dress himself without assistance but as his 'chorea' appeared to improve, William stated he had purposely feigned being worse than he really was at the time he attacked the asylum doctor. In fact, his intention had been to rob the doctor of his key and make good his escape – William also confessed he falsely stated he was suffering from gonorrhoea, adding he had a wife and ten children living at home. The conclusion of Medical Staff was that whether or not William had made these confessions on account of his insanity, there did not appear to be 'the slightest doubt' that a great amount, if not all, of the chorea William claimed to be suffering from had also been feigned – nevertheless, William continued to have a shower bath every day except Sundays and 'some Mondays'. As the muscular difficulties associated with his chorea appeared to ease, the shower baths were temporarily discontinued in order to determine whether the apparent improvements made in his gait were maintained. By May, however, William's behaviour was becoming increasingly disruptive again as he had now started 'slashing' at his bed every night – on one occasion cutting his right hand on the edge of the bed, requiring an application of 'linseed poultice' to the wound he had inflicted upon himself.

Poor Health

By the end of the month, the wound on William's hand had not healed – it was now inflamed and, in fact, it appeared to be getting worse as the inflammation extended to the palm; the wound was therefore lanced on the 29th May and 'muriate tincture of iron' applied three times daily. Despite William's attempts to interfere with the dressing, an improvement was noted over the next few days – although it was still found necessary to make another incision in the hand and to repeat the course of treatment. This time, a 'locked glove' was placed on William's hand to prevent him from removing the dressing – a method of restraint that proved effective as the 'erysipelatous' inflammation soon abated. By 8th June, however, a boil on William's left wrist had emerged and the inflammation on his right hand was now extending up the length of the arm and from which an abscess was starting to form. A few weeks later, the hand was described as much improved with the 'openings' on the arm appearing to heal up. On the 4th July, great concern was expressed over the state of William's digestive system because of his 'disinclination to eat suitable food'. This was exacerbated by William's tendency to 'swallow anything disgusting' whenever he had the chance, causing him to badly suffer from diarrhoea. William refused any medicine 'whatsoever' to alleviate his symptoms, under the impression it would poison him. The following day, on 5th July 1878, the diarrhoea had disappeared but William himself remained very weak and 'wandering in his talk'. William was ordered a tablespoonful of whisky mixed with water every hour but whilst this revived him a little, William continued to sink and he died at 6.05 pm of what was described as 'chronic mania and erysipelas'.

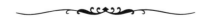

JAMES SMITH

Date of Admission: 14th October 1878

Background

32-year-old James worked as a 'Travelling Linen Draper' (Salesman) and lived with his brother, Edward, in Bath Lane Terrace, Newcastle; for a week prior to his admission, James had been 'annoying' the priests and pianists of nearby St Mary's Church. Having arrived outside the church, James would then sit or kneel by the roadside with his hands folded and eyes closed as if absorbed in prayer, taking no notice of his surroundings or the people around him. It was only with some difficulty that James could be made to reply when someone eventually approached and questioned him – only stating he had been praying 'almost since birth' before adding he 'hoped he might have enough learning to become a priest'. The night before his admission, the concerned priests at St Mary's had only contacted police after James – in an excited state – refused to get up from the pavement and go home. When the police arrived, James refused to co-operate, resisting so much they were obliged to lift him up and carry him off to the police station.

Admission

On admission, James was noisy and in a state of 'religious exaltation', only managing to sleep through the early part of his first night in the dormitory of Ward Six. At about 4.30 in the morning, James became so excitable and violent he was removed to a single room for his own safety. At 10 o'clock that morning, James was lying quietly in bed when he said to an attendant he wanted to speak to a Father Ryan 'at once' as he was dying. James was subsequently prescribed a sedative and a draught of chloral hydrate to be given at bedtime in order to settle him and to help him sleep. At first, James refused all medication and meals, saying he would take nothing until 'Father Ryan' was brought to him – he soon acquiesced, however, and within the week, he was 'up and out' with the other patients. Over the next few months, James became more settled and able to occupy himself usefully as a ward helper, despite occasionally displaying signs of a 'disposition to be dangerous'.

Turbulent and Dangerous

By April the following year, James's mental condition had improved and he continued to be gainfully employed on the ward but by November his mental state had deteriorated again. For the next year or so, he remained largely unchanged and James was generally inclined to be 'turbulent and dangerous' towards others. James was now spending most of his day in 'garrulous chatter', but despite this, he was able to remain in employment although by this time, it meant working outside in the gardens. At the beginning of 1882, there was 'no diminution' of James's excitability, having now developed an 'exaggerated sense' of his own importance; he continued in a state of 'maniacal excitement' over the next two years. Despite such behaviour, James still managed to continue working and by May 1884, was even helping with 'the carts' over at the farm. In 1886, James was becoming increasingly obstinate and stubborn in manner as he laboured under the belief he was being persecuted by others who wished to do him harm. James was still employed outdoors, but now he often became unsettled and excited, invariably taking offence against what was said to him and refusing to go out to work. Over the next few years, James's general demeanour continued to fluctuate in this way, and he remained unpredictable and very changeable in both mood and behaviour.

At times, James would be bright and cheerful and state he was very happy, whilst at others, he could be 'querulous', hurling abusive language as he accused and insulted everyone around him. When happy and contented, James would continue to work outside with others – even although he was still liable to sudden excitable outbursts during which he could be violent and abusive. Throughout 1890, James remained generally free from such excitable behaviour, but nevertheless remained susceptible to disturbed episodes – especially if 'thwarted' or contradicted or whenever his grandiose delusions were challenged. Over the next few years, James continued in a state of 'chronic mania with partial dementia', occasionally joining in with the 'associated amusements' enjoyed by the other patients. Regardless of his mental state, James remained in fair physical health and despite a 'slow, labouring heart', continued to work outside in the gardens. By 1894, James was still working outside every day – even though he remained 'untidy, abusive and incoherent' and 'full of grandiose delusions'.

Very Rambling

James suffered some deterioration in his physical health in 1895 and was therefore given employment indoors despite his general untidiness and eccentric behaviour – as well as his noisy and abusive manner. Throughout that year, James continued in poor health and remained 'peculiar' in his general conduct; his mental state at this time was described as having 'no decided change in any respect'. James's physical condition gradually improved and the following year he appeared in much better health, so much so, he was now assisting in the housework of the ward and – despite his delusions of exaltation and 'very strange manner' – also put to work in the Attendants' Mess Room. Over the following few years, James's mental state remained unchanged and he continued to be untidy, restless and excitable, often rambling incoherently in his conversation. His delusions persisted – now, he called himself 'Master of the World' – and he remained generally childish and eccentric in his behaviour. Despite such conduct, however – and apart from his underlying heart condition – James remained in fair physical health and, as he 'gave no trouble', continued to work well in the Attendants' Mess Room. By 1900, James was showing no 'alleviation mentally' and although he could be 'stupid, restless and excitable', over the following years he ate and slept well and remained merely 'quietly peculiar'.

Indifferent Health

From 1905, and for the following few years, James worked – despite his silly and childish ways – in the kitchen adjoining the Attendants' Mess Room, and remained in fair bodily health. In July 1908, James decided he had had enough of working in the Mess Room and refused to continue working there; instead, he returned to working in the gardens – only to be 'usefully' put to work again in the kitchen of Ward 8 in 1909. He was still working in the kitchen in 1910, but by April of that year, James was recovering from an attack of influenza from which he made slow progress but never quite regaining his previous good health. In May, James was suffering from oedema of the feet and was therefore put to bed where he made some improvement; over the following months, however, there was no particular change to his general physical health which remained largely 'indifferent'. On 30th November 1910, James 'looked ill' and was put to bed; his heart sounds were noted to be feeble with an associated weak pulse and for which he was given a 'heart tonic mixture'. On the morning of December 1st, James was pale and breathless; considerable oedema of the feet was evident and he appeared much weaker. James showed no signs of improvement at this time, and his condition deteriorated throughout the day. At 5.10pm that evening, James died after having suffered from pneumonia in conjunction with mitral heart disease.

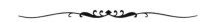

JOHN DICK

Date of Admission: 30th September 1880

Background

John was a 42-year-old Presbyterian Scot who worked as a joiner and lived with his wife, Wilhemina, in Ramshaw Street, Newcastle. For the past three months, John had been 'melancholic, desponding and tired of life'; he was also refusing to eat as he suspected his wife of trying to poison his food. John had previously been under care at this asylum where he had remained for eighteen months, only being discharged in November of last year (1879).

Admission

When admitted, John was 'eccentric and mysterious' in his conversation and wore a furtive, suspicious expression when speaking as if not to divulge what was actually on his mind. John laboured under the impression he was being persecuted by the Roman Catholic authorities who, he believed, had conspired with others to have him admitted to the asylum. John nevertheless quickly settled in and was otherwise quiet and orderly in his behaviour; by the end of the first week, John was 'usefully occupied' in the joinery shop. His 'mental excitement' and suspicious nature, however, became increasingly prominent over the next few weeks to the extent he was unable to continue working there. Over the next year or so, John maintained a furtive demeanour and 'dogged, reticent manner' – interspersed with sporadic outbursts of maniacal excitement and disturbed behaviour. By April 1882, John's – increasingly frequent – excitable outbursts meant he was often thought to be 'dangerous' as he charged around loudly preaching and using threatening language; in doing so, John would gesticulate extravagantly to emphasise the point he was trying to make. Over the next two years, John remained as 'dangerous as ever' and was inclined to walk about in an excited manner. Sometimes, he would preach for an hour at a time at the top of his voice but at other times, John became quiet and 'moody, sullen and morose' in manner. Despite this unpredictable behaviour, and although there was no improvement in his mental state, by October 1884, John was working outside in the grounds with other members of the gardening squad.

Cannot Engage in Conversation

By May 1885, John was still working in the gardening squad despite there being no reduction to the intensity of his mental excitement – an example of this being the 'heated sermons' he frequently preached to imaginary audiences. Around this time, John was asked how old he was, to which he replied: 'I do not let anyone know my age and the only time I shall do so will be when the attorney signs a 'testamentation' in my favour for a large sum of money'. Despite now working as a ward helper, John's circumstances changed little over the next few years and he continued to be 'silly and apt to be noisy' in his general behaviour with an inability to engage in any meaningful conversation. By January 1890, the only real change in John's circumstances was his re-employment in the joinery shop – now though, he persisted in entering a room backwards, the intention being, he declared, to keep Scotland on his right-hand side so as to 'more efficiently defend it'. Throughout the early 1890s, John remained eccentric, had an aversion to conversation and easily became agitated and abusive towards others – although such conduct did not prevent him from continuing to work in the joinery shop. Whilst John had always enjoyed reasonable physical health, it was now noted he was suffering from arterial degeneration and hypertrophy of the heart. This was a condition, however, that did not alter his delusional thoughts and 'peculiar manner' as highlighted by his continued defence of Scotland – only now he was 'quiet and gave no trouble' in attempting to do so.

Works with Joiner

From 1895, and over the next few years, John continued in fair physical health in spite of his heart condition. Nevertheless, his behaviour – now described as 'very eccentric and grotesque' – had deteriorated as he became increasingly aggressive and quarrelsome if anybody disturbed him. Still working in the joinery shop, John could be 'peculiar and secretive' and become agitated if obstructed; his delusions persisted and he often refused to speak to anyone although when he did, he rambled incoherently. John remained 'very irrational and strange in conduct' and by March 1900, was still considered to be 'very deluded'. Although in fair physical health, John continued to have intermittent problems with his heart condition but otherwise remained 'restless, threatening and aggressive' over the next few years.

Apart from suffering a large abscess on the back of his left wrist in January 1904 which soon healed, John's health remained fairly robust, and despite his strange and eccentric manner he was still fit enough to undertake work on the ward. By July 1908, however, and although still 'peculiar in conduct', John's physical health was starting to decline as his heart condition became more evident; throughout the rest of that year, John remained in poor general health. By April 1909, and although still 'very deluded and eccentric', John was becoming increasingly feeble. By September, his heart was described as very weak and he was confined to bed. John rallied somewhat in October and began to improve a little, he had regained his appetite and was now noted to be 'back to his usual self'. At the beginning of December, John suffered a relapse and his condition deteriorated throughout the rest of that month. On the morning of 25th December, he became very cyanosed and breathless and at 3.40pm, John died of cardiac degeneration.

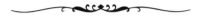

JOSEPH ROUTLEDGE

Date of Admission: 25th April 1885

Background

Joseph was a 40-year-old shoemaker who lived with his wife, Emma, in Nelson Street, Newcastle. For the previous two weeks Joseph had been behaving strangely and talking incoherently in conversation, boasting about his wealth and influence and stating that he was involved in a 'maze of difficulties'.

Admission

On admission, Joseph was rational in his answers when asked simple questions about himself and his family but quickly adopted a 'noisy and aggressive attitude' in response to threats he felt were being directed against him by 'unseen agents'. At times, Joseph talked in a rambling and 'utterly unintelligible manner' about a day of reckoning and the judgement that was about to be bestowed on him. Joseph was immediately assigned a single room and kept in isolation because he suffered from scabies and acne and for which sulphur ointment was applied twice daily. Over the next few days, Joseph exhibited delusions of persecution and conducted long conversations with imaginary people, insisting his communication with this 'unseen world' was real – a world revealed to him, he stated, because his knowledge was of a 'superior kind'. By May the following month, and still in isolation, Joseph's scabies slowly improved though he continued to excitedly pursue imaginary conversations with others – conducting them in an authoritative voice, whilst waving his hands around. At such times, Joseph often made long, rambling statements such as 'I return to my home like a lamplighter, a lamplighter has to do with chastisement, I have to do with chastisement, my skin affliction is the result of the milk of human kindness, chastisement has to do with the reckoning of the milk of human kindness'.

Over the next few weeks, however, Joseph showed a steady improvement and was allowed out into the airing courts to associate with other patients despite the threat he was thought to pose to those around him. By the beginning of July, Joseph was again subject to outbursts of maniacal excitement, during which he indulged in 'long, loud and incoherent harangues to imaginary individuals'. Such behaviour meant Joseph could often become pompous and overbearing in his attitude and general demeanour, stating for example, that he could not sleep well at night unless 'God Almighty warmed the blankets' for him.

Converses Excitedly

Over the next few years, Joseph continued to suffer from outbursts of maniacal excitement on a regular basis, his face becoming flushed and his 'conjunctivae suffused' as he proceeded to shout and pray loudly. At other times, Joseph often became 'absurdly pompous', adopting an 'extravagant and fantastic' demeanour as he used 'abusive and filthy' language to get his message across. Although such periods of 'silliness' invariably passed, Joseph's continued rude and aggressive behaviour meant he was still apt to be a danger both to himself and to others. By 1890, there was no noticeable improvement in Joseph's circumstances and his conduct continued to be 'boisterous and aggressive'; by the end of that year, however, he had been free from 'active excitement' for three months and was therefore able to undertake some work on the ward. Over the next year or so, there was no change in Joseph's condition and although noisy and excitable, he continued to help out on the ward – until August 1892, when he started to become increasingly 'idle and quarrelsome'. Such disruptive and aggressive behaviour continued into the following year, highlighted by an incident on the afternoon of 10th May 1893, when Joseph made good his escape whilst out in the grounds with a working party. Nothing was heard of Joseph for two days until he was brought back late at night, having been found 'wandering about in town'. Despite his tendency to idleness, and his delusional, excitable and quarrelsome behaviour, Joseph was still able to work on the ward – his eccentric and aggressive manner notwithstanding.

Little Change

Joseph's condition remained unchanged over the next few years and whilst he was now less excitable and able to work in the cobbler's shop at his previous occupation of shoemaker, in November 1896, he was still being described as 'quarrelsome and abusive, noisy and incoherent'. Such behaviour continued into 1897 with Joseph rambling in his conversation as he expressed his thoughts on 'many strange ideas and fancies'. One of these may have led Joseph to make another escape attempt on 27th October, when he disappeared from the cobbler's shop into the early morning fog that pervaded the grounds that day. He was soon brought back – 'none the worse for his journey' – by the police, who had found him wandering about Jarrow in the early hours of the following morning. Apart from this episode, Joseph continued as before in his strange and eccentric manner – presenting with excitable and quarrelsome behaviour for the next year or so. Apart from his mental state, Joseph had always enjoyed good physical health but during the night of 22nd August 1899, he was noted to have passed about a pint of blood via his rectum and became very 'collapsed and pale' although no cause for the haemorrhage could be ascertained at the time. Joseph remained on bed-rest for the next few weeks and whilst he still suffered from a few small haemorrhages from the bowel, he was deemed to be not as anaemic as he had been before. Joseph continued in his recovery and by 10th November he was once more up and about – even though he remained 'pale and haggard' in appearance.

Strange and Eccentric

By the beginning of 1900, Joseph was still acting in a strange and eccentric manner and he continued to ramble in his conversations. In April, he was put on bed-rest suffering from severe anaemia due to the frequent haemorrhages emanating from his bowels. This was caused, it was now determined, by Joseph's 'constant interference and manipulation' of his anus during defecation; around this time, it was also noted he was 'probably masturbating frequently'. Despite remaining anaemic, Joseph's physical health had improved by July and he was soon up and about working on the ward again. Joseph's chronic mania, however, continued to render him 'excitable quarrelsome, and aggressive' and although he ate and slept well and continued to do a little ward work, mentally, he was 'quite unchanged in every way' over the next few years. Throughout 1904 and 1905, Joseph remained excitable and, at times, aggressive, grumbling discontentedly and picking fights with those around him. In January 1906, Joseph displayed a hard, dry cough and was put to bed after becoming feverish; nothing was detected in his lungs although it was suspected he was suffering from heart disease. Throughout February, Joseph ate very little and he became noticeably thinner, anaemic and weaker. In March his condition gradually declined and whilst no abnormal signs could be detected in his lungs, he was still coughing a great deal. By the end of March, Joseph was becoming increasingly feeble and his only nourishment was provided by drinks of milk. On the morning of 1st April,

Joseph was in a semi-conscious condition and he was now unable to accept any nourishment at all. Upon examination, Joseph's heart sounds could not be heard, he was almost pulseless and it was felt that he was gradually sinking. The following morning Joseph was found in a 'moribund condition' and died at 10.15am, apparently of heart disease and pulmonary phthisis.

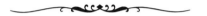

THOMAS CAVERHILL

Date of Admission: 28th January 1887

Background

Thomas, a 44-year-old widower with one daughter, was a 'Waterman' by occupation, who suffered from epilepsy; at the time of his admission,

Thomas was residing at the Union Workhouse in Newcastle. After having a seizure, Thomas would usually suffer a loss of memory and appear dazed and confused – alternatively, he could become excitable and violent, believing that people were plotting against him. According to the Master of the Workhouse, Thomas was 'violent and unmanageable, unfit for the imbecile ward here'.

Admission

Thomas conversed rationally and coherently when admitted, answering such questions as were put to him and his general health and bodily condition were considered fair. Nevertheless, Thomas was regarded as being of unsound mind with his powers of memory, judgement and attention severely impaired. According to Thomas, he was subject to epileptic seizures about once a fortnight and experienced 'petit-mal' episodes as often as once or twice a day. Thomas settled in well over the following week but on the 4th February he fell off his chair during a seizure – his first attack since being admitted. In falling, Thomas's face came in contact with the edge of a form (bench) and he sustained a deep, three-inch laceration to his left cheek which caused profuse bleeding. After coming round from the seizure, Thomas became 'extremely excited and dangerous' which made it difficult for staff to treat his wound and meant he had to be restrained 'by means of a camisole' before being strapped to the bed with sheets. This then allowed staff to insert a 'dressing plug' into the exposed wound and apply pressure to stem the flow of blood; once Thomas settled, the plug was removed and a light dressing put in its place. Thomas slept well that night and appeared 'quite composed' by the following morning – both eyelids, however, were now swollen and oedematous with the left eye 'much bruised'. After a week, the wound had almost healed and by the end of February, Thomas was 'cheerful and well-conducted' and making himself generally useful around the ward.

Querulous and Irritable

Over the following few months, Thomas remained 'polite and obliging' and apparently free from any epileptic seizures; he talked sensibly and continued to be gainfully occupied as a ward cleaner. During this period of stability, Thomas was still 'apt to excitement' and would often become querulous and complaining during such episodes. On the 25ᵗʰ October, Thomas fell to the ground suffering from a seizure and sustained a wound over his right elbow which was then treated with carbolic acid oil. A few days later, an abscess formed on the elbow joint from which 'about an ounce of pus' was released. The wound didn't respond to being treated with a linseed poultice and a considerable amount of swelling remained, causing the arm and forearm to become oedematous and aggravating Thomas enough to make him 'exceedingly querulous and irritable'. In December, complications set in as boils developed on the forearm, for which Thomas was ordered an iron mixture, but after taking the first dose he refused to take it again, saying he didn't need it. By January 1888, the forearm had healed sufficiently, helping to calm Thomas down to the extent he started making himself useful again – his 'usual querulous tendency' now in abeyance as he maintained a bright and cheerful disposition. At the end of May, however, Thomas fell after suffering another seizure and injured his right arm once more; the injury was left untreated this time due to his lack of co-operation – he did, however, tolerate keeping the arm in a sling until it improved some weeks later. Thomas was subject to more epileptic seizures over the coming months during which he frequently injured himself, but he still managed to keep his job as a ward helper – a job he continued to hold over the years despite his susceptibility to seizures and the injuries they often caused.

Thomas suffered around sixty seizures in each of the following two years – many of them at night – and he remained 'very subject' to attacks of petit-mal during which he was frequently abusive and inclined to be irritable and garrulous. By the end of 1891, Thomas was still working on the wards but was now complaining of constant headaches due to the frequent attacks of petit mal he experienced and for which he sometimes took potassium bromide – only to refuse his medication as soon as he started to feel better again.

Frequent Epileptic Fits

Thomas, who was now thought to be labouring under chronic mania, was suspicious of others, believing they were conspiring against him and out to cause him harm. Thomas had frequent periods of excitement when he could be 'querulous and hypochondriacal' but generally, he was cheerful and 'quiet and civil as a rule' – when not having seizures.

Throughout 1892, Thomas had a total of one hundred and twenty-three seizures – forty-eight during the day and seventy-five at night – but by 1897 they had become less frequent in number although they remained both 'slight and severe' in their presentation. Despite the debilitating nature of his seizures and in spite of occasional periods of bed-rest for such ailments as bronchitis and lumbago, Thomas remained in fair bodily health – even continuing in his job as a ward cleaner. Although the seizures were now infrequent, Thomas remained restless, bad-tempered and childlike after experiencing them and often complained of ill-treatment by staff who came to his assistance. Thomas's hypochondria also meant he constantly complained of various ailments – usually imaginary – which often left him tearful whenever he came round from a seizure. Thomas remained concerned about his health over the coming years, often grumbling discontentedly and complaining of dizzy sensations and the injuries he invariably sustained – usually caused as Thomas suddenly fell to the floor during a seizure. In May 1899, he was left with a limp after painfully damaging his knee and in May 1901, he fell against a chair badly cutting his right ear, badly bruising the same ear again in November 1906.

During these years, Thomas remained very childish in manner and conversation, he took no interest in his surroundings and would periodically burst out into episodes of excitement. The chronic nature of his epilepsy and the frequency of his seizures often left Thomas in a weak and exhausted condition, frequently confining him to bed and unable to take any nourishment. On 25th August 1908, Thomas had six 'very heavy' seizures throughout the day, seven more during the night and a further six by 8.30am the following morning. By 1st September, Thomas had had fifty-nine more seizures; he remained on bed-rest over the following two months as the seizures had been continuing very much on a regular basis. Despite the decline in his health, Thomas was often restless and noisy but as time went by, he became increasingly exhausted and feeble. Thomas had seven 'very heavy' seizures during the night of 18th November; on the morning of 19th November 1908, and in a much debilitated condition, he had seven further seizures. Thomas deteriorated through the course of the day and he died at 7.05pm that evening.

WILLIAM AINSLEY

Date of Admission: 5th July 1888

Background

William was19-years-old and had been in the workhouse in Newcastle for three years. According to his sister, William had fallen on his head when he was only a few weeks old but otherwise, he was just like any other boy up to the age of twelve – since then, however, he had become 'bad-tempered and stupid'. During his time in the workhouse, William had generally been excitable in nature, often talking in a loud voice as he prayed for salvation in the belief he was about to die. At 11pm the night before he was admitted, William was 'suddenly seized' with this fear of dying and started praying and shouting – he refused to settle down and persisted with his prayers in a state of 'religious exaltation'.

Admission

William appeared 'thin, untidy, wet and dirty' when first admitted but quickly settled down, before lapsing back into a period of 'excitement and stupidity'. It was felt that William was of 'unsound mind', indicative of which was his expectation the ward doctor would 'bring him the horses' on which he intended to ride races in London. Over the next few days, William constantly asked about his racehorses and would express his satisfaction when told they were to arrive shortly. William continued to entertain delusions about his ability as a jockey – if shown a newspaper, he would randomly point to a paragraph and state it contained a report of the last race he had won. On one occasion, William pointed to pictures of horses hanging on the walls of the ward and said – 'with glee' – his racehorses had arrived at last. William generally exhibited a quiet and cheerful nature and tended to laugh immediately whenever being addressed – such a disposition was very changeable, however, as he was also inclined to bouts of aggression during periods of excitement during which he was apt to smash the ward windows.

Dirty and Fatuous

Physically, William was in fair condition and by April 1889, he had been working for some time as a ward helper or outside in the gardens. His mental state, however, remained very much the same; he would laugh without any apparent cause and he could be 'silly' in his general behaviour. By April 1891, William's physical health had declined, although he was still able to help out around the ward or sometimes even work outside. Now, however, William was being described as 'dirty and fatuous' and thought to be labouring under dementia. Over the next few years, William generally remained 'untidy, noisy and incoherent', but when free from excitement he was very quiet, seldom spoke and generally regarded as being 'dull and stupid'.

Throughout the second half of the 1890s, William's behaviour remained unchanged – he could be excitable and quarrelsome in nature and continuously grimace as he muttered to himself. Despite his eccentric conduct, William's physical health had improved again and over the next few years, he continued to either work outside in the gardens or on the farm. By April 1904, however, William was refusing to eat and, as he started to lose weight, his physical health began to decline once more. On 20th May, William was put to bed where his condition improved slightly – only to deteriorate again a few days later with the onset of a troublesome cough and 'night sweats'. Although feeble and still confined to bed, William rallied slightly and he started to take a little nourishment. By 2nd June, however, his health deteriorated once more and he gradually became worse as he perspired freely, coughed frequently and was unable to sleep. Over the following weeks William was kept comfortable although by now, milk was his only nourishment. On 14th August 1904, William had had a bad night and at 10.30 the following morning, he passed away having suffered from pulmonary phthisis.

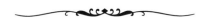

WILLIAM MCALLISTER

Date of Admission: 22nd November 1888

Background

William was a 46-year-old publican from Jesmond, Newcastle. He had been married for twenty-six years, his wife describing him as a very quiet man who only got excited 'after drink'. William had always drank heavily and for the past two years, had been in a state of chronic alcoholism without having received any treatment. Around a year previously, William had been ejected from the bar – owned by his mother-in-law – which he had been managing for nineteen years, after a family dispute. This had greatly affected William and he became 'very despondent'; for the past three months, he had also started having epileptic-type fits and was becoming increasingly restless and excited. According to his wife, William would laugh and cry without any apparent reason and sometimes try to get out of the house, occasionally hitting out at her in his attempts to do so.

Admission

On admission, William's speech was quite unintelligible, he was noisy, restless and he appeared 'frightened at nothing'. Over the next few days, William could be 'vacant and silly' in his general demeanour but also apt to be quite noisy and aggressive to those around him. William had difficulty in understanding what was said to him and sometimes acted in a 'stupid and depressed' manner. At other times, he became 'excitable and suspicious' in his behaviour. William's mental state improved slightly the following month as he quietened down and regained his 'powers of articulation', which meant he could now occasionally enter into a reasonable conversation.

Despondent and Lachrymose

Early in 1889, William frequently entertained the delusion he was in heaven and was inclined to become 'despondent and lachrymose' when the mood took him. As a rule, however, William was more disposed to be generally content and although his gait was inclined to be unsteady and his speech impaired, William was able to occupy himself by doing a little 'light work' around the ward. Through the course of that year, however, William's general demeanour was regarded as one of being 'stupid and vacant' and that he was deemed to be of only limited intelligence.

In January 1890, William's physical health was noted to be declining and that he was also 'degenerating mentally' as he became easily dejected and would start weeping without any apparent cause. Over the following few months, William alternated from being 'fairly cheerful' in outlook to suffering bouts of depression and despondency – despite this, William still managed to carry out helping out around the ward. William's mental condition remained much the same during 1891 with his physical health now being described as only 'fair' because of his varicose veins and the intermittent heart disease that had now been diagnosed. The exhibiting of symptoms such as impaired gait and slurred speech, which had been attributed to what was now thought to be his 'General Paralysis', were also becoming increasingly noticeable. Otherwise, William was generally regarded as 'quiet and industrious' and his circumstances remained largely unchanged as he 'cheerfully' worked fulfilling his duties as a ward cleaner – interrupted only by the occasional episode of depression. Over the following few years, however, the symptoms associated with William's general paralyses were becoming increasingly apparent. Nevertheless, he remained generally 'happy and demented' during this time and despite suffering the impediments of slurred speech and unsteadiness on his feet, he was still capable of helping out on the ward. Although usually good-tempered as a rule, William still remained 'emotional and irritable, childish and forgetful' at times. The next few years saw William's physical health gradually decline further as he began to lose weight and became 'feebler' in his gait, making it more difficult for him to get around.

Indifferent

In January 1901, William was described as childish but 'pleasant to con-verse with' although the general paralyses he suffered from, meant he was regarded as more of 'a dement'. By 1903, and seemingly quite indifferent to his surroundings, William nevertheless appeared quite happy and contented. He was still regarded as something of a good worker and was employed in the kitchen of Ward 6 even though his physical health continued to gradu-ally decline. By 1905, William was now doing very little in the way of work because of his general ill-health; his mental state was also increasingly poor as he was observed continually talking to imaginary people. Over the next year or so, William's health deteriorated further and in August 1907, a small growth – 'about the size of a pea' – thought to be an epithelioma, was identi-fied under his tongue. By September, the growth was becoming larger and William now had difficulty in swallowing, which resulted in his physical health deteriorating even further. The epithelioma continued to increase in size and by October, William was only managing to swallow soft food. By November, he was becoming more feeble as the epithelioma continued to grow and by January 1908, William had been confined to bed for quite some time; he now became increasingly weaker as the epithelioma got bigger.

A few months later, William's deteriorating health was further compli-cated by his heart condition and on 25th October, 1908, he gradually sank and died at 11pm that evening, of cancer of the tongue in conjunction with cardiac degeneration.

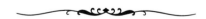

WILLIAM BEST

Date of Admission: 21ˢᵗ May 1894

Background

William, a 50-year-old painter, had started drinking heavily when his wife died eight years previously. For the last five of these years, William had begun to stay in bed all day, taking no interest in anything except ensuring his 'personal wants' were met. William's son, also called William, and daughter Barbara, had become increasingly concerned as they saw their father's condition deteriorate over the six months prior to his admission. William would lie in bed – his 'bed and apparel in disorder' – and take no interest in anything, expressing no anxiety as to how he was 'maintained and from whence' and his bed had a 'urinous odour'.

Admission

William was admitted in a dishevelled state, his long hair hanging down over his neck and his dark beard and whiskers all matted and dirty. He had a sallow complexion, defective teeth and patches of psoriasis all over his back; at 5 feet 8½ inches in height, William weighed only 6st 6lbs. Appearing wholly indifferent to his circumstances and untroubled by his situation, William instead seemed rather pleased with himself and talked in a boastful way about his abilities and 'dirty habits'. Despite 'sudden paroxysms of noisy and abusive excitement', William submitted quietly to being bathed and having his hair cut before he was assigned to Ward Three to sleep in the Infirmary Dormitory where he was kept under constant observation.

Paroxysms of Excitement

William became quieter and better-behaved throughout the month of June with his physical health also showing some improvement despite his thin physique and pale complexion. Over the next few months, however, William continued to be untidy in appearance and susceptible to occasional 'paroxysms of excitement' when he would become childish in manner. By the beginning of 1895 William was quiet and cheerful again – although he still thought highly of himself and persisted in having a great opinion of his own abilities. William's faith in himself gave him the confidence to sing at the patients' weekly dance – 'dreary lengthy songs of his own composition'. His evident self-worth was apparent to others as he continued singing his 'dreary' songs for the rest of that year – regardless of how they may have been received. When not singing, William tended to ramble in his conversation and whilst in fair physical health, it was thought his mental condition suggested evidence of general paralysis despite no 'definite corroborative physical signs'. Although William could be 'very weak-minded and childish' in his behaviour, throughout 1896 it was unable to mask the symptoms – such as disturbed gait – of his general paralysis which were now thought to be more 'marked'. Over the next few years, William continued without any significant change in his condition, but he was nevertheless regarded as being of a happy disposition and generally quiet 'as a rule'. William was held in high esteem as a good worker and helped out with ward duties even although his general paralysis now made him increasingly unsteady on his feet – particularly in cold weather.

Gave No Trouble

From 1900, and despite his defective memory, William remained unchanged; he could be silly and childish in manner on occasions but was otherwise mainly 'quiet and obliging', giving no trouble as he helped out around the ward. Over the next few years, William's circumstances remained much the same, although now he could be restless and 'foul and abusive' in conversation whenever he was in a talkative mood. By this time, William's physical health was also beginning to fail; on the morning of 3rd November 1904, he suffered a 'syncopal attack' in the bathroom, from which he made a quick recovery by the 'dinner hour'.

By 1907, and despite periods of excitement, William was generally quite content; in March of that year he had another syncopal attack, this time a severe one during which he lapsed into unconsciousness. William was put to bed and hot cloths applied to his extremities before being given some brandy – actions that prompted another prompt recovery. The following week, however, he had another attack and he was put back to bed again – but once more, he was up and about soon after. As a result of these attacks, William became increasingly hypochondriacal and continually maintained he was going to die, noisily and abusively stating he was about to 'peg out'. Early in 1910, William was diagnosed with heart disease and, upon receiving the news, was convinced his death was imminent. For much of that year, William remained in a fair condition but on 4th August, he was noted to be 'not looking so well' and sent to bed; by October, he was considerably improved and was allowed 'up daily' from his bed. Over the next year, William's physical health improved again and he suffered no more symptoms of ill-health – this, however, did not reduce his hypochondria and the feeling he was the victim of an 'unjust law'. Consequently, William became very unhappy – and often threatening in manner – at not being taken seriously about the claims he made regarding how poorly he felt. Indeed, his remarks could be 'dry and caustic' and he appeared to take some pleasure in being 'abusive and vituperative' when discussing his symptoms.

By April 1912, William had lost weight and was now in a 'feeble and bodily-reduced condition' – a state that did not prevent him from being foul-mouthed and abusive to others. Over the next two years, William's health fluctuated greatly, although it remained 'generally poor'. On 5th January 1914, William became ill again and he was put to bed on a milk diet with a daily dose of 2ozs of brandy which helped him to improve over the following week. William's health declined again on 4th March after suffering an attack of bronchitis; he was once more sent to bed and given a cough mixture, put on another milk diet and, this time, given 8ozs of whisky daily. By 1st April, William's bronchitis was clearing up and he was breathing a little easier. On 15th April, however, and believing he saw objects on the ceiling, William became very restless, noisy and talkative during the night. Towards the end of April, William was becoming gradually weaker and his mind was starting to wander; by June, however, and despite being very weak, he showed signs of considerable improvement. Nevertheless, William's health deteriorated again and by 12th December, he alternated between being 'very heavy and torpid' and periods of restless delirium. On 24th December, William was 'quite helpless' as his condition deteriorated further; on 31st December 1914 William died of heart disease at 4.55am.

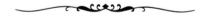

JOHN TINDALL

Date of Admission: 24th May 1894

Background

John, a 47-year-old 'repairer of telegraph wires', had been married for twenty-three years and lived with his wife and child in Byker, Newcastle. In September 1892, John had fallen forty-two feet, sustaining a head injury and breaking both legs; according to his wife, John had never been well since. For two weeks prior to his admission, John had been harbouring delusions of suspicion, felt his food was being poisoned and that people were plotting against him. He elaborated by stating: 'they want to put me in a prison. I have seen people watching me about. They get into my house; I have heard them between the roof and the ceiling. They put something in my food. This morning I thought two men were putting a bundle of wire in my yard to say I had stolen it, I went to the police station'.

Admission

On being assigned to Number 3 Ward John was described as 'stout but flabby and in rather shaky bodily condition'. He wore a blank expression as he walked to the ward with a 'rather ataxic gait' before quietly submitting himself to being bathed. It was thought John had symptoms suggestive of general paralysis, but apart from his gait, 'want of expression' and a 'slight trembling of the lips and tongue', further potential signs appeared to be masked. John didn't speak much of his delusions but he remained suspicious of others and still felt people were still trying to poison him which, as a result, meant he was inclined to eat very little; otherwise, John gave no trouble and spent his time 'quietly playing dominoes etc'. After a few days John seemed a little brighter and stated he didn't hear the voices quite as often; an improvement to his appetite was also subsequently noted. Despite remaining 'quiet, cheerful and orderly' over the next few months, John's delusions nevertheless persisted, and he continued to see and hear imaginary people whom, he stated, still conspired to poison his food. Now, however, they featured less prominently and John tended to eat and sleep well. Despite having a poor memory – he couldn't recall whether he was married or not – and some concerns over the symptoms of his general paralysis, John remained quiet and cheerful and gave no trouble. By December, however, John's mood became increasingly changeable as his delusions of suspicion had started to escalate and he became more 'fanciful' in his thinking as a result. He frequently complained and became more convinced than ever that people were out to harm him by poisoning his food.

Many Delusions

In January 1895, John's delusions had, for the last few weeks, led to him becoming more and more excitable in both mood and behaviour. On 7th February, this resulted in him being fed by oesophageal tube after he had refused to eat for three days. John was fed via this route for a few more days before he started to eat independently again and reverting back to his usual 'quiet, cheerful dementia'. John remained convinced his food was still being poisoned, however, and that chemicals and electricity were now acting on him as well, causing him to experience 'strange sensations'. On 20th June, John was put to bed after vomiting and suffering from 'hot skin, constipation and dark, scanty urine', where he remained for about ten days – taciturn in manner and passively obstinate. Having recovered, John was once more quiet and cheerful as his delusions slowly subsided – but, for the rest of 1895, whenever the feelings of persecution – wrought by 'unseen agencies' – overwhelmed him, John refused to eat and he lapsed back into his usual excitable and aggressive behaviour.

Throughout 1896 and 1897, John was described as 'quiet, cheerful and rather lethargic' when not distressed by his delusions – but 'very troublesome' when he was. Under their influence, John was often surly, abusive and threatening, especially if he was being bothered – such as when intervention was required to feed him by tube due to his persistent refusal to eat 'poisoned' food. Despite such beliefs – and methods – persisting over the previous few years, John was still described as being 'stout and in good health' – even although his delusional beliefs now started to include the poisoning of his clothing as well as his food. In February 1898, John pulled his bed to pieces, and attempted to burn his clothes in an effort to get rid of this poison. Over the next few years, John was often hostile, surly in manner and abusive as he continued to struggle with his delusions of persecution. John was generally reserved 'as a rule' when his delusions were in abeyance and he often refused to engage in conversation, but when any intervention was required, John could be abusive and threatening in both language and conduct. By 1903, and over the next few years, John showed no change to his behaviour 'in any respect'. He could be very reserved and seldom spoke, taking no interest in his surroundings whilst remaining liable to outbursts of excitement during which he was often regarded as aggressive and dangerous.

Throughout the following years, John remained much the same but was still in good, general physical health apart from complaining of pains in his legs from time to time. In April 1909, John developed a carbuncle on his left cheek which was dressed with a 'fomentation' four times daily; however, it got larger over the next few days as the inflammation spread around his left eye. On the morning of 24th April, an incision was made in the carbuncle, allowing a large quantity of pus to be discharged with a further large quantity of pus discharged a few days later. However, John developed a high temperature and his health started to decline; on 1st May, John's condition suffered a marked deterioration and John died at 7.15, on the evening of 4th May 1909, as a result of the carbuncle on his left cheek with associated cardiac failure and congestion of the lungs.

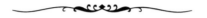

HUGH BEGG CLARK

Date of Admission: 4th June 1894

Background

42-year-old Hugh was a wood turner who lived with his wife, Annie, in Heaton, Newcastle. Three years previously, Hugh had been admitted for six weeks to Morningside Asylum in Edinburgh because of his heavy drinking. Since then, Hugh had been healthy and strong until almost two years ago when he fell 20 feet in an accident from which he never made a full recovery. For the past four months, Hugh had been drinking 'immoderately' again and for the last week he had become agitated in behaviour and suspicious in manner. Hugh would often ramble in his conversation, making comments such as: 'two men who looked like private detectives have got influence over me by electricity or hypnotism. They whisper in my ears with wires and draw my history out of me. People spit in the street with derision as they pass me by, thinking me a sodomist. They are moved by animal magnetism or electricity. There is a class of people about, practising hypnotism. It will kill me if you look at my heart, at the post mortem you will find it shattered'.

Admission

Hugh was shaky and tremulous when admitted with a livid complexion and a 'somewhat dazed expression', he talked incoherently on a variety of subjects that often related to electricity and how it could be used. Hugh was suffering from delusions of persecution and believed he could see and hear imaginary people who accused him of crimes he hadn't committed and conspired to 'work on him with batteries'. Over the next few days, Hugh remained in a restless and agitated state, eating little and sleeping badly at night. By the end of June, Hugh had settled down, although he still found it difficult to sleep because of the hallucinations he experienced. Hugh now acknowledged these hallucinations were caused by drink, but he still adhered to his delusional beliefs, especially ones where people were out to get him and to annoy him with 'electricity and telephones'. The next few months, however, saw Hugh slowly improve physically as he started to regain his appetite and sleep better. Although Hugh's delusions were less prominent, they still persisted and he continued in his feelings of persecution where imaginary people were trying to harm him. By the end of 1894, despite such thoughts and occasional episodes of excitable restlessness, Hugh became 'cheerful and industrious', his general health slowly improved and he was able to converse intelligently 'on most points'.

Brought Back Drunk

In the first few months of 1895, Hugh continued to experience delusions of persecution although now, some doubt existed as to whether they were feigned or not, in view of his otherwise generally cheerful disposition. Hugh was inclined to order the younger attendants about and was 'fond of his own way', even managing to get a job working in the gardens despite being regarded as a 'rather lazy' individual. Hugh took full advantage of this occupation as, on more than one occasion, he would make his escape from a working party without being seen – often coming back 'considerably the worse for drink'. On one such occasion, in March 1895, Hugh escaped from a working party and was brought back drunk, after which he remained morose and 'rather sullen' for some weeks. Over the next five years, Hugh's delusions of persecution persisted but generally, he was usually 'reserved, silent and suspicious in manner'. At other times, however, Hugh was bright and cheerful and – now considered a good worker – continued to work outdoors despite his reputation for trying to escape; at the weekly dances, he was even considered to be an 'energetic dancer'. Hugh could still be unpredictable in his behaviour, as exemplified on 14th November 1898 when he was sent by the attendant in charge of his working party to collect some tools from a shed, which Hugh took as an opportunity to escape. When he didn't return, the attendant thought Hugh was sheltering from a shower of rain that had just come on and his disappearance was only discovered when the rain subsided. The following day, Hugh escaped again and was brought back by an attendant from Newcastle quayside just as he was boarding a boat bound for Leith in Scotland.

Continually Grumbling

From 1900, Hugh remained in general good health and whilst he could be quiet and well-behaved, there were also times he would be restless and excited. On such occasions, Hugh was inclined to complain, constantly grumbling as he voiced his suspicions about those around him. He continued in his job working outside in the gardens and, by 1904, was considered to have remained 'quite unchanged in every way' – indeed, Hugh was still trying to make his escape at every opportunity, doing so again on 30th September – although this time he came back of his own accord after only an hour.

Over the following years, Hugh became lazier and attempted to do as little work as possible, with periods of indifference often punctuated by episodes of suspicious excitement. As a result, Hugh was now regarded as someone who was 'very peculiar'. His suspicions and threatening manner tended to make him childish and quarrelsome – behaviour attributed to the delusions of persecution he continued apparently to experience. On 19th September 1910, Hugh suffered from a bout of diarrhoea, which he appeared to have recovered from after a few days. A few months later, however, Hugh was looking somewhat thinner and a decline was noted in his general health. On 27th January 1911, Hugh vomited after a 'syncopal attack'; investigations into his condition subsequently revealed he had thickening of the arteries. Over the following months, and despite periods of childish behaviour and rambling conversation, Hugh's physical health improved – before deteriorating again. In October, he was once more in poor physical health and looked 'reduced' as he had lost weight and suffered from recurring bouts of diarrhoea. A slow improvement in Hugh's health slowly followed, although he remained thin and 'not robust'; nevertheless, he continued to work – but this time, inside, working on the ward. On 5th May 1912, Hugh was sent to bed after vomiting 'copious fluid material' and undigested food for which he was given a 'bismuth and pepsin mixture'; a belladonna plaster was also applied over his abdomen. A few weeks later, Hugh was feeling a little better, his appetite had improved and he was able to get up out of bed for a short while. By 10th July, however, Hugh was back in bed again after vomiting and complaining of stomach pains – appearing to believe he had to undergo the 'torture' of his discomfort for some obscure reason which he hinted at but refused to discuss. He remained in bed and continued to experience severe attacks of stomach pain and regular episodes of vomiting. On this occasion, deep palpation of his abdomen revealed the presence of a lump. By 8th August, Hugh was in a 'much reduced state' and taking very little nourishment; he was very weak, suffering from a troublesome cough and evidently in pain. Hugh was getting weaker daily, and at 6.45pm on 17th August 1912, he died, apparently of a malignant disease of the stomach.

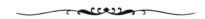

WILLIAM REED

Date of Admission: 13th December 1895

Background

William, a 30-year-old porter, had been married for six years and had two young children; he had always been healthy but had been experiencing epileptic seizures since around the time he got married. At first, the fits were 'regular but slight' then gradually they became more intense in nature. Over the week leading up to his admission, William had suffered a series of fits which left him increasingly 'passionate and excited', culminating in causing him to violently shake his wife as he threatened to 'do for her'. William's actions meant his wife was now afraid to live with him and, fearing for the safety of herself and their children, had called for the police. William was excitable, restless and 'absurd in manner' when taken to the workhouse in a condition of acute mania.

Admission

William had no recollection of having been brought to the workhouse and had no idea how long he had been there – it could have been 'days or weeks'. It was soon decided to admit William to the asylum; as he was being transferred, William stated, with a dazed expression, he was epileptic and would often fall down in the street without warning. William only remembers there was a fire somewhere and that he was crying to God for mercy when he saw his parents among the flames; it was noted, however, that both of William's parents had been dead for a number of years. In a 'dazed and stupid' manner, William arrived at the asylum and walked quietly to Ward Three to be admitted, where he was 'bathed without trouble'. William could give no account of himself with regard to recent events but quickly settled in over the next week, free from the seizures he had been experiencing before his admission. On 20th December, however, William suffered three seizures during the day, followed by two more that night. A further four seizures were experienced the following week which left him confined to bed in a 'restless and excited condition'. William was still being confined to bed at the beginning of 1896 despite remaining in a state of general restlessness. Indicative of this, on the 3rd January he managed to tear the skin off his nose by pushing his head between the pads of the padded room in which he was currently sleeping. Over the coming months, however, William became quieter in manner and brighter in mood despite averaging a seizure approximately every three days, after which he would become a little depressed for a short time; William only had nine seizures during the month of June but for the rest of 1896 they declined even further in frequency. William remained in good general health but often complained of 'numerous fancy ailments' – he also began to suffer episodes of mania and periods of excitement during which he could be 'aggressive and violent'.

Aggressive and Spiteful

Over the next few years, William continued to experience seizures and although they occurred at 'longish intervals', they were severe in nature and would often leave him 'stupid, dazed and irritable'. After such episodes – described typically as an 'epileptic mixture of the religious element' – William would become emotional and irritable, sitting down to write religious letters that were sometimes 'mixed with abuse'. At times, William could be impulsive and spiteful, resulting in an incident on one occasion in April 1899, when he colluded with three other patients to make a 'concerted attack' on the attendants in charge of a working party. No injuries were sustained by those involved in the incident but for some time afterwards, William remained 'quarrelsome, disagreeable and hypocritical'. Such disruptive behaviour continued throughout much of 1900; in February, he incited other patients to stop working and to escape, in March he punched one patient on the mouth – only to do the same again the following day to another patient. Both attacks were unprovoked with William denying he had struck either man.

Over the next few years, William settled down and had periods of being quiet and generally well-behaved – these periods of relative calm were noted to occur when he was not prone to having any seizures. However, William remained liable to 'outbursts of noisy excitement' when he could become 'very quarrelsome, troublesome and interfering'. By the end of 1903, William had been 'free from excitement' for some months and had remained so, despite the discomfort of suffering a large abscess on the back of his neck; on 9th January, 1904, the abscess was excised and a 'large quantity of pus' released. The cavity was subsequently packed with cyanide gauze and rapidly healed well. By 26th January, William had been suffering seizures daily for the previous six days and consequently, he became quarrelsome and restless and continually made accusations and allegations against other patients. On the morning of 30th January, William complained of ill-treatment by one of the attendants; a few days later he struck another patient whilst out in the airing court and when an attendant went to separate them, he too was attacked. William and the attendant quickly got into a struggle, falling and getting up from the asphalt three times before his colleagues eventually came to the attendant's assistance whilst William was offered assistance by two of the other patients. The only evidence of the incident having taken place was a large bruise on William's back.

Quiet at Present

For the remainder of 1904, and for the following year, William was generally 'quiet, well-behaved and free from fits' – although at times, he continued to be 'excitable and restless, threatening and abusive'. From 1906, William began once more to experience seizures with increasing regularity. Between August and November of that year, he had twenty-four, and between November and January 1907, he experienced a further forty-five. As a result, William suffered frequent periods of excitement during which he became abusive and threatening in such a manner it often caused him to be 'mischievous and interfering'. Over the next few years, this cycle of behaviour continued, as periods of quiet behaviour were interrupted by episodes of restlessness and aggression – usually following one of his seizures, which were now averaging twelve a month.

By January 1911, William's seizures and recurring periods of aggressive excitability were making him increasingly difficult to manage as he believed himself to be persecuted and 'wronged' by those around him. William remained suspicious in manner over the following months with his behaviour continuing to lack any degree of control. By January of the following year, William started to show signs of deterioration in his general physical health – exacerbated by the severe epileptic seizures which he continued to experience. Although still inclined to be excitable and aggressive at times, William remained in poor bodily condition throughout much of 1912. On 28th December, William was noted to be 'not so well today' and was sent to bed, although physical examination had shown 'nothing definite'. William was put on a fluid diet and prescribed 'spirits of ammonia' but by 4th January 1914 William had grown considerably weaker and was now 'apt to wander in his mind'. William deteriorated further through the following day and night. He died at 6am on 6th January 1914, apparently of lobar pneumonia.

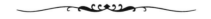

JOSEPH HOPE

Date of Admission: 17ᵗʰ May 1897

Background

Joseph was a 24-year-old single man who lived with his parents in Mitford Street, Newcastle. He had always been in good health until contracting typhoid fever about sixteen months prior to his admission. Four months after recovering, Joseph decided to become an ironmonger and went into the hardware trade – a venture that proved unsuccessful as, after only eight months, Joseph was deemed to have 'failed in business'. His first attack of mania had started around the same time with Joseph stating 'my mind travels with other people's minds' in the belief he knew what they were doing and thinking. For the previous six months, Joseph had thought this ability to read minds and understand the reasons for people's actions meant he himself no longer needed to work, believing his powers now gave him 'ample means' with which to live. Joseph would often see people he imagined were present and who, he felt, were watching and following him around and conspiring against him. During this period, Joseph would often excitedly ramble in his conversation but for the previous three weeks, he had started to become violent towards his father – seizing him by the throat on one occasion.

Admission

On admission, Joseph mumbled incoherently in conversation as he attempted to express his thoughts and 'exalted' ideas. Nevertheless, Joseph gave little trouble, although the delusions about his 'thought transference' were quite evident. Over the next few months, Joseph continued in good general health and despite his childish manner, he was regarded as 'very quiet and orderly'. Being of a settled disposition, Joseph was now able to help out around the ward even though he continued to exhibit the delusions he experienced on admission, writing 'long letters' about them to his parents.

Idle and Listless

Towards the end of 1897, Joseph's delusions still featured prominently and appeared to cause him some distress as he periodically took to standing about in 'strange attitudes, making queer gestures' – at other times, however, Joseph could be 'very quiet, idle and listless'. By February the following year, Joseph was once more troubled by his delusional beliefs and although he denied experiencing them, they appeared evident in his strange manner and behaviour. Joseph showed no improvement through the remainder of 1898 and whilst he could be childish, he was nevertheless able-bodied and so was put to work with a gardening party. Throughout 1899, Joseph was untidy and apathetic, his memory proved defective, he was rambling in his speech and unable to converse rationally. Joseph's eccentric behaviour continued over the next few years and it was thought he was slowly becoming more demented. At times, this could lead to Joseph becoming restless and aggressive in his behaviour, whilst at other times, he was generally more settled, quiet and well-behaved. By the end of 1904, Joseph was still working outside in the gardens, but otherwise, his mental state remained 'unchangeable in every way' – as highlighted by his usual rambling and incoherent conversations.

Periods of Excitement

By 1905, Joseph could be noisy and abusive and was described as someone who showed himself to be 'demented and stupid' with no change of any kind in his circumstances. By February 1906, however, Joseph's periods of excitement were becoming less frequent and for much of that year he was generally quiet and well-behaved. The following year saw Joseph's behaviour decline once more as he became increasingly abusive, aggressive and more difficult to manage. This behaviour continued largely unchanged over the next two years or so, but on 20th February 1910, Joseph was observed to be 'not so well', having lost his appetite and found to be suffering from a high temperature. On 23rd February Joseph was diagnosed with lobar pneumonia and his condition gradually deteriorated over the next two days. At 8.50 on the morning of 25th February 1910, 37-year-old Joseph died of pneumonia following a short period of influenza.

Male Case
Histories:
Photographs

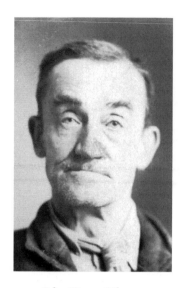

John Henry Gibson:
Admitted 7th July 1874

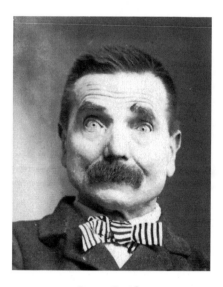

James Smith:
Admitted 14th October, 1878

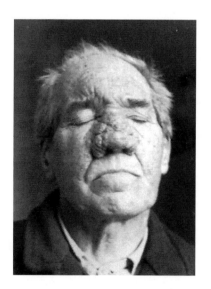

John Dick:
Admitted 30th September 1880

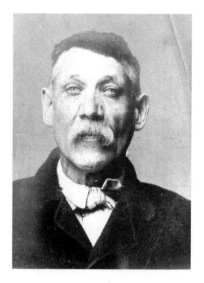

Joseph Routledge:
Admitted 25th April 1885

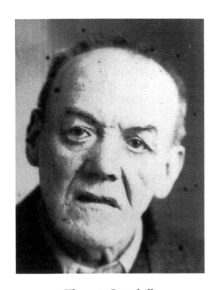

Thomas Caverhill:
Admitted 28th January 1887

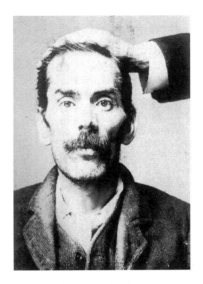

William Ainsley:
Admitted 5th July 1888

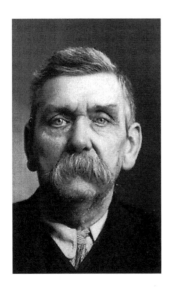

William McAllister:
Admitted 22nd November 1888

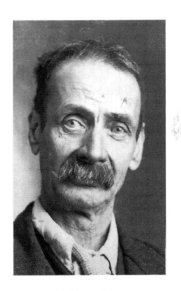

William Best:
Admitted 21st May 1894

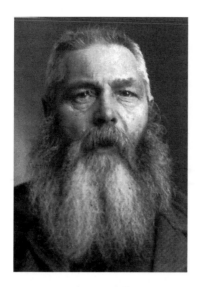

John Tindall:
Admitted 24ᵗʰ May 1894

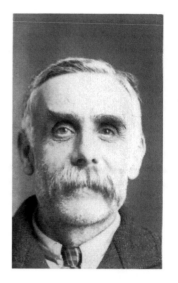

Hugh Begg Clark:
Admitted 4ᵗʰ June 1894

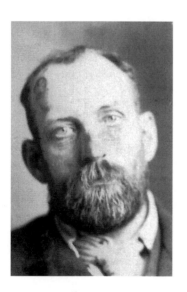

William Reed:
Admitted 13ᵗʰ December 1895

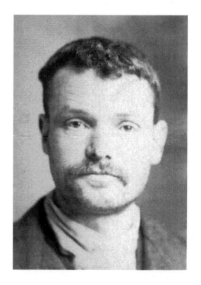

Joseph Hope:
Admitted 17th May 1897

Female Case
Histories:
Photographs

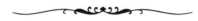

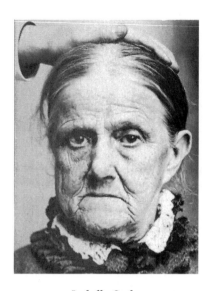

Isabella Stult:
Admitted 15ᵗʰ April 1873

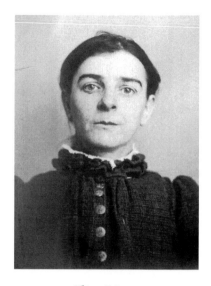

Eliza Dixon:
Admitted 17ᵗʰ August 1894

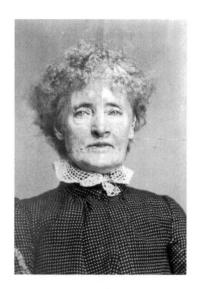

Jane Dalglish:
Admitted 14ᵗʰ May 1897

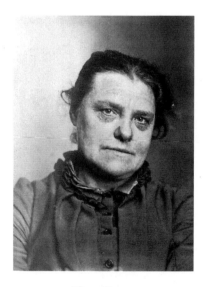

Mary Young:
Admitted 17ᵗʰ March 1900

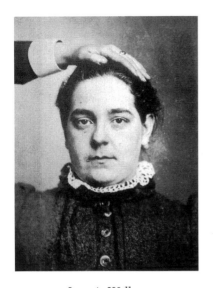

Jeannie Walker:
Admitted 27ᵗʰ March 1903

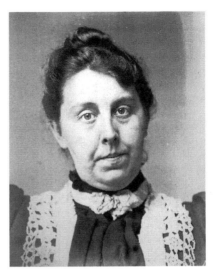

Jane Scott:
Admitted 7ᵗʰ November 1903

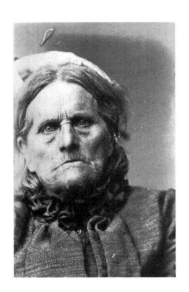

Emma Hadley:
Admitted 5ᵗʰ January 1904

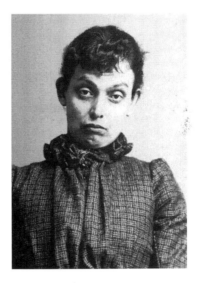

Eliz. Jane Kirkup:
Admitted 9ᵗʰ January 1904

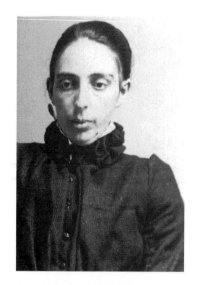

Georgina Mathews:
Admitted 16th April 1904

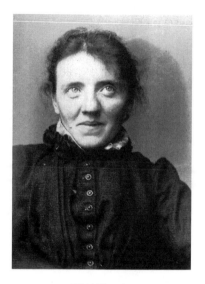

Alice Howitt:
Admitted 27th May 1904

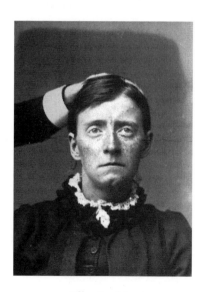

Ellen Lackie:
Admitted 3rd June 1904

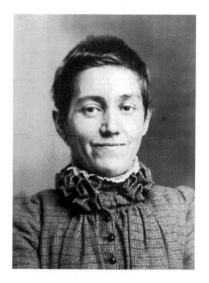

Louisa Robinson:
Admitted 10th August 1904

Female Case
Histories

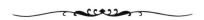

ANNIE BUCKLEY ALIAS SMITH

Date of Admission: 18th March 1886

Background

Annie was a 23-year-old single girl living in Ord Street, Newcastle with her partner Reuben Smith, a brass furnisher whom she had known for about two years. Her illness – attributed to childbirth – had lasted for eight days prior to her admission when Reuben first noticed Annie's mind was starting to wander and she was unable to sleep. According to Reuben, Annie had previously showed no signs of distress and had coped very well with her period of confinement which had started on 5th March. Annie had always enjoyed a good appetite and had been attentive to her personal appearance but by the 16th March, she was eating very little and neglecting herself. The day before her admission, a neighbour had observed Annie with the baby in her arms and squeezing it so tight 'as to hurt it' and saying she wanted to poison it.

Admission

On admission, Annie displayed a strangeness of manner and made statements such as 'I have to suffer for the whole world. I have done wrong to everybody. Eh, I am a bad one, am I not? I shall clash my brains if only I had forgiveness. I would lie down and die, there is an explosion to go off all over the world'. Annie was assigned to the Second Ward of the Female Division to sleep in a padded room and to be visited every hour by the night nurse. Annie did not appear to be aware of her surroundings and stared vacantly ahead, making little effort to reply to any questions put to her. Although in fair bodily condition, Annie's general state of health was described as 'very bad' – her abdomen was hard and rigid; both breasts were slightly enlarged and no milk exuded from the nipples when pressure was applied between finger and thumb. The following day, Annie was described as 'somewhat improved' even though she was refusing any attempt to persuade her to eat. At 10am that morning, Annie was given a pint of beef tea administered via a nasal tube. This procedure was repeated again at noon when Annie was given an egg whipped in milk along with a 'little emulsioned castor-oil'. Over the next few days, Annie found it difficult to settle and slept poorly at night, but appeared much brighter in mood the following day. Although seemingly incapable of engaging in conversation, Annie was inclined to sing 'snatches of hymns and songs' to herself whenever she became excited.

Puerperal Insanity

By the following week, Annie was still refusing to eat or drink properly, causing her tongue to become very dry and coated with a thick, yellow fur. As she persisted in this refusal, Annie continued to be fed by the 'mechanical means' of a nasal tube – even though she occasionally vomited some of the feed back up. Annie was visited by her partner, Reuben, later in the week who was subsequently informed Annie continued to express delusions of personal identity – a condition thought to have resulted from 'puerperal insanity' arising from the recent birth of her baby. By the end of the month, Annie began to show some signs of improvement as she started to answer questions and accept food in the form of milk. By April, Annie's bodily condition had slowly improved to the extent she was now able to walk around the ward, although her delusions of personal identity were once again becoming increasingly prominent. As such, Annie was still inclined to be 'very silly' and had no idea where she was or to whom she was talking. When asked a simple question she would only repeat the statement 'I don't know what to say'.

Whilst continuing to comprehend very little of what was put to her and despite no apparent improvement in her mental state, over the remaining few months of 1886 Annie's physical health underwent a marked improvement. Annie was now able to undertake a little needlework and sewing in the workroom, but she nevertheless remained incapable of entering into a conversation with anyone and generally kept quietly to herself. Annie's mental state and general behaviour remained largely unchanged at the start of 1887 and she continued to be 'extremely silly' on occasions. By May, Annie was still occupying herself with needlework and tended to smile vacantly whenever she was spoken to – but never replying to even the simplest question. Despite her silence, Annie was now deemed to have made sufficient progress and, on 31st August 1887, she was discharged as recovered.

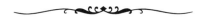

NO.	NAME.	SEX.	AGE.	SOCIAL STATE.	OCCUPATION.	RELIGION.	EDUCAT
157	Ann Knight	F	28	Single	Steam loom weaver	Ch. of England	

Previous History of Case.	*This unfortunate creature has been the victim of a seducer who after child in person. She had to leave her employment and when she was and her child drew its nourishment from her as sole. She much may performed.*

DURATION OF DISEASE.	CAUSES.		FORM OF INSANITY.
	MORAL.	PHYSICAL.	
6 months	Desertion of her lover after giving birth to child	Lactation v. starvation	Melancholia .

found she was pregnant by him immediately left her to bring forth her her relatives to whom the burden the herself lived on as little food as possibl be easily imagined she became weak in body and mental derangement

ANN KNIGHT

Date of Admission: (No Date Specified) December 1866

Background

Ann, a 28-year-old factory worker, was described as an 'infatuated creature and the victim of a seducer' – one who had immediately left her after finding out she was pregnant by him. Now unemployed and having to bring up the baby on her own, Ann had been living with relatives but since being deserted by her lover six months previously she had become increasingly 'melancholic' and ate very little. The shock of her circumstances, it was felt, could 'easily be imagined' and this, along with her 'mental derangement' and poor diet made her physically unwell and unable to lactate sufficiently in order to provide nourishment for her baby.

Admission

On admission Ann intelligently answered questions in a 'hollow and manly' voice and gave a fair account of herself, but she nevertheless seemed dull and depressed and took no interest in anything happening around her. Insufficient nourishment, distress at having her child taken away and the subsequent drain on her system had left Ann anaemic, thin and 'much exhausted'. Soon after her admission, Ann was prescribed an iron mixture, 'good food' and 1 pint of porter daily.

Melancholic Dement

Ann's condition was described as that of a 'melancholic dement' and it was feared she would not improve or recover from her circumstances. By the end of December 1867, the principal characteristics of her condition were noted to be apathy and indifference, highlighted by a lack of interest in her surroundings. Throughout 1868, Ann continued to present as apathetic in manner and generally inclined to exhibit a 'sulky, sullen disposition'. Nevertheless, Ann seemed content within herself and appeared to accept the situation she found herself in, even taking up regular employment working in the laundry; in doing so, her general disposition and circumstances remained much the same over the next few years. By 1873, however, Ann's physical health was failing a little but despite this she continued working, this time on the ward even though she continued to appear 'very depressed' in her manner. Throughout 1874, Ann worked hard at keeping the ward dormitory tidy but, in going about her duties, she was often inclined to be very irritable in mood and could not bear any interference. Ann remained in poor physical health but there was nothing 'especially noticeable' regarding her current circumstances and despite her irritable nature she never complained – if left alone – and rarely even spoke.

Complaining Disposition

At the beginning of 1875, Ann was working in the South Dormitory when she took it upon herself to explain to a member of staff that she originally came from Stockport where there were boats. When asked if there was any water for them to sail upon she kept her head bent down, cast her eyes to the ground and replied she didn't think there was any water there. Apart from this isolated episode, Ann continued to speak infrequently and, in June of that year, was removed from the First to the Third Ward on account of her quiet disposition – as well as, now, her untidy habits and poor personal care. A few months later, however, and in a departure from her usual silence, Ann began to adopt a 'very complaining disposition', particularly about her food, which she would often grumble about loudly and violently. This behaviour continued for the next few months before Ann reverted back to her usual quiet persona. Despite now regarded as being quite demented, she continued to be a 'very useful' ward helper who enjoyed attending Divine Service and the occasional Wednesday Dance.

Persecuted by Evil

The following year, in April 1876, Ann complained she could not sleep at night on account of something being concealed in her pillow. Ann believed this was related to her being persecuted by evil in the form of young men who were out to harm her. Over the next two years there was no improvement 'at all' in Ann's mental state although she did manage to continue working on the ward by assisting nursing staff in carrying out their duties. By April 1879, a positive change was noted in Ann's behaviour as she became increasingly inclined to take notice of the events happening around her. This slow improvement was maintained throughout the following year with Ann continuing to occupy herself as a ward helper – but by April 1881, her mental state started declining again as she once more became indifferent to her surroundings and seldom spoke. On 29th April 1881, however, and over fourteen years after her admission, Ann was discharged as 'not improved'.

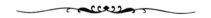

ISABELLA STULT

Date of Admission: 15ᵗʰ April 1873

Background

41-year-old Isabella, the wife of a labourer from Hawes Street, Newcastle, had recently been complaining of flashing lights and 'peculiar feelings in the head'. For the past two weeks Isabella had been unable to sleep at night, feeling that she had brought harm on all connected with her and that she was 'eternally damned'. According to her husband, Isabella often sat up in bed through the night 'talking and pointing with her fingers', claiming she could see such things as horns glowing bright red at their tips.

Admission

Anaemic, emaciated and in poor physical health, Isabella appeared 'melancholic' and unable to comprehend the questions put to her. Over the next few months Isabella gradually became physically stronger but nevertheless remained depressed, rarely getting up from her chair where she sat in a 'low, melancholy state'. By November, a pair of 'locked gloves' had to be put on Isabella's hands to prevent her from constantly picking at her skin; sometimes, she even had the 'revolting and brutal tendency' of eating her own flesh. The following months saw Isabella wearing the locked gloves continuously but even so, it was only with some difficulty she could be restrained from either irritating the sores on her skin or from attempting to remove the surgical dressings that covered them.

By February of 1874 – and throughout that year – some improvement was gradually noted in Isabella's behaviour, although her mental state remained largely unchanged. Accordingly, Isabella did not have to wear locked gloves all the time and was now to be found usefully occupied in sewing 'for the greater part of the day' – she was, however, still required to wear locked gloves at night for her own safety. In 1875, Isabella started picking and eating her own flesh again, which meant she had to once more start wearing locked gloves all the time; even when temporarily removed, Isabella would immediately start picking at the skin. Apart from a few days in August when she briefly stopped her 'disgusting habit', Isabella – despite close supervision – succeeded in injuring herself by picking at her neck and shoulders whenever the opportunity presented itself. Over the next two years, the severity of Isabella's attempts at self-injury fluctuated, although when well, Isabella attended Divine Service and sometimes even the weekly dance. Usually, however, Isabella was inclined to sit with her knees drawn up to her chin and mutter to herself.

Disposed to be Dangerous

Isabella's depressed state continued unabated in this way for some time, but by October 1880 it showed signs of subsiding. By April the following year, Isabella was 'exhibiting a tendency to more cheerfulness' – a tendency that could still develop into over-excitement, when she was 'disposed to be dangerous' towards herself and others. By May 1884, a slight improvement was noted in Isabella's mental state, although she could still be 'very querulous' and inclined to complain a great deal for no apparent reason. The general improvement in Isabella's mental state continued into the following year so that by April 1885, she was working as a ward helper and taking more of an interest in what was going on around her. Even so, Isabella remained very quiet and showed a disinclination to enter into conversation with anyone.

Isabella appeared to become very demented over the next few years, incapable of replying to even the simplest of questions and was regarded as being in a state of 'absolute fatuity'.

By 1890 – and for the next few years – there was no discernible improvement or change to Isabella's demented state and she was still liable to attacks of 'aggressive excitement'. In August 1894, Isabella was described as 'demented, untidy and occasionally dirty in her habits', inclined to idly sitting around all day muttering incoherently to herself – sometimes making the 'peculiar noise' of croaking like a frog. In April 1897 and despite exhibiting delusions of persecution, Isabella was transferred to the Farm Ward where some improvement was noted to her general health. There, Isabella was not quite so listless and became a little neater in appearance and more orderly in her habits. Nevertheless, Isabella developed a belief that the man who visited the Farm Ward to regulate the ward clocks was, in fact, her husband who had come to the Farm to visit her. Isabella continued in good general health into the following year although a deterioration in her mental state was noted early in 1899 as she became increasingly incoherent in conversation and frequently made unintelligible grunting noises.

Defective Memory

In February 1900, Isabella left the Farm Ward and was transferred to Ward One where, for the rest of that year, she rambled in her talk and continually expressed delusions of persecution and convinced that people were going to harm her. Isabella constantly expressed fears she was on the male side of the asylum and shouldn't be where the men were – her confusion compounded by the fact that the ward she now resided in used to be a male ward prior to the recent enlargement of the asylum. Over the next few years, Isabella's circumstances remained much the same, with her general conduct now regarded as being 'merely eccentric'; her physical frailty, however, was becoming increasingly evident – a factor that did little to dampen her 'peevish and querulous' manner.

On the morning of 20th February 1906, Isabella was sent to bed after complaining of diarrhoea and sickness. By 24th February, Isabella was averaging around ten bowel motions over a twenty-four hour period. These motions were noted to be very foul as they contained some blood and slime as well as a 'very disagreeable odour' that was now starting to emanate from her. Two days later, Isabella was transferred to the nearby Isolation Hospital as she became increasingly frail and unable to take any nourishment; by 1st March, Isabella's health was declining and although she rallied briefly, 74-year-old Isabella died from colitis at 10am on 2nd March 1906.

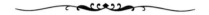

WINIFRED MALAN

Date of Admission: 6th July 1869

Background

Winifred, a 38-year-old single woman of 'very limited intelligence', was regarded as incapable of anything but the simplest of domestic duties. She had recently given birth to an illegitimate child who had since been placed in the workhouse. It was thought Winifred's present 'maniacal attack' had been brought on by anxiety during her recent period of confinement.

Admission

On admission to Newcastle's temporary asylum at Bensham in Gateshead, Winifred was incoherent and excitable as she wandered restlessly around, weeping at the loss of her new-born child. Over the next few months Winifred's condition gradually improved and she was soon engaged in regular employment, undertaking work of the 'most simple kind' – whilst still liable to 'capricious and quarrelsome' outbursts in her general behaviour. This behaviour changed little during the next twelve months and, having now been transferred to the new asylum in Coxlodge, she remained quite excitable and unpredictable at times, which often rendered her dangerous towards others. Winifred's circumstances remained largely unchanged over the next few years and when settled, she would quietly work in the sewing room or kitchen – Winifred was, however, still liable to periodic episodes of excitement, which usually lasted about a month at a time.

Disorderly Conduct

During one particularly violent outburst of excitement – on 9th August 1874 – Winifred became very abusive and aggressive as she proceeded to break windows and strike out at nursing staff. Winifred quickly became 'quite unmanageable' and so was taken to her room to be given a hypodermic injection of '¼ grain of acetate of morphia', which had the desired effect of calming her down. Over the following few months Winifred remained settled, becoming quiet and 'very useful' in the work she undertook helping out on the ward. Bouts of erratic behaviour continued, as highlighted in the first few months of 1875 – during one period in February, for example, Winifred was well-behaved and quietly helping out by working on the ward, but soon after had to be removed from the weekly dance for 'disorderly conduct' whilst dancing. Furthermore, on 24th April several articles belonging to the asylum were found concealed in her room and subsequently removed

– amongst them were two bowls full of broth, about which Winifred had become 'very excited'. Other disruptive episodes followed and on 3rd May, Winifred hit another patient with her shoe; she also became very violent at teatime a few days later by attempting to throw a basin at someone. Not long after these incidents, Winfred bit the thumb of yet another patient when both were outside in the airing court. When involved in such altercations, Winifred frequently used the most 'disgusting and indecent' language as she assaulted her fellow patients, invariably kicking out at nursing staff who would rush to intervene.

Winifred's disruptive behaviour continued unabated and on 2nd June, she accused nursing staff of mistreating her, showing the ward doctor various cuts and bruises on her right leg and hip as evidence of this. Upon further enquiry, it was discovered Winifred had refused to undress at bedtime the night before and when the nurses tried to remove her clothing, she 'kicked them right and left', striking one of them severely in the stomach. In her frenzy, Winifred had slipped off the bed and fell against it, causing the injuries she had shown the doctor. The following day – and without a moment's warning – Winifred 'sprang upon' the Head Nurse, spat in her face, seized her by the hair and pulled a clump of it out, which caused an 'effusion of blood' beneath her scalp. It was only with great difficulty that the ward doctor – who happened to be doing his rounds at the time – and two nurses were able to rescue the Head Nurse from Winifred's grasp. The incident resulted in Winifred being placed in seclusion overnight. This measure, however, only had a limited effect as at dinner time the following day, Winifred threw a bowl at the heads of two nurses and tried to 'bite, scratch and kick' both of them. With the assistance of a doctor who had been summoned, Winifred subsequently received a 'shower bath' which helped calm her down. Shortly afterwards, Winifred produced a portion of the Head Nurse's hair she had torn out the previous day and presented it to the ward doctor, accusing the nurses of having pulled it from her own head. It later emerged this had been the 'second or third' time Winifred had practised this particular deception as she was known to sometimes collect all the loose hair she could find and make similar accusations against one of the other patients – or any nurse who happened to be on duty.

'Covered with Bruises'

For the rest of June, Winifred made her presence felt and became a 'focus' for complaints directed against her from almost everyone else – the ward doctor even exclaiming he could hear her 'all over the house' owing to the amount of noise she tended to make. Winifred would often be 'covered with bruises' on her legs and arms – the result of her own aggression as she frequently required three or four nurses to hold her down whenever she needed to receive any medication. By the end of June, Winifred had become more subdued and, over the next few months, was starting to show some signs of improvement in her general behaviour. October, however, saw another deterioration as Winifred gradually became more excited and inclined to, yet again, annoy those around her. Despite this, Winifred was not yet considered particularly dangerous; she was currently 'clean in her habits' and as such, attended Divine Service on Sundays and went along to evening dances on a Wednesday. Winifred, however, could still become very jealous of any little favours granted to other patients such as when they were granted parole. On the morning of 17th November, Winifred became very excited and started a fight which resulted in her being given a draught of chloral hydrate to calm her down; she was given another draught at bedtime which helped her to get at least six hours' sleep – this proved so effective, another draught of chloral hydrate was administered every night over the next few weeks. Night-time draughts of chloral hydrate were given less frequently from December onwards as Winifred was now managing to sleep quite well without them. Although she started to become more co-operative with nursing and medical staff, Winifred was still a risk to her fellow patients, often quarrelling with them and sometimes even throwing them against the wall. Winifred eventually showed some signs of improvement by March 1876 but was unable to sustain it; on 12th May, Winifred was given an injection of morphia to quell her excitement after becoming 'very disorderly' in the Dining Hall.

Pretending

Over the next few weeks, Winifred was often given a morphia injection for disruptive behaviour, its effects usually helping to keep her quiet through the course of the day. On the 20th May, Winifred picked a fight with another patient and sustained a bloody nose and bruised cheek which resulted in yet another morphia injection. On 26th May, after becoming excited, Winifred was yet again given an injection of chloral hydrate but this time it only caused her to become 'helplessly drunk' afterwards. Winifred's excitable behaviour persisted throughout June and into July, often resulting in the administration of draughts of morphia in order to help keep her behaviour manageable. Such a course of action was usually only effective for short periods at a time, however, and would invariably be followed by violent outbursts – such as the incident which occurred at bedtime on 11th July when Winifred broke several panes of window glass. In the morning, she broke several more panes and was subsequently given an injection of chloral hydrate. That night, however, Winifred proceeded to yet again smash the glass of more windows. Her disturbed behaviour was now seriously escalating as in addition to such episodes of destruction, Winifred was also attacking some of the other patients – even injuring one of the nursing staff, then pretending to suffer from an epileptic fit. Another morphia injection was given. This particular injection appeared to have had the desired effect as Winifred's behaviour was now described as 'perfectly quiet' for the rest of the day – evidence of the morphia's effect showing in the contracted pupils of her eyes. Winifred remained settled over the next few days, only becoming excited at intervals when she would wander around the ward 'dancing, singing and shouting' – which inevitably led to a morphia injection being given to quieten her down. This pattern of behaviour continued over the next few months; in one incident on 4th September she was given a dose of castor oil after an episode of 'excitement and violence' which she proceeded to spit into the eyes of the doctor administering it, causing him intense agony. Following this incident, however, Winifred 'continued to improve each day' and by the end of September she was being described as 'quiet and industrious'. Such behaviour did not last too long as, on

8th October Winifred became excited during Divine Service which resulted in her removal – once more – back to the ward where she 'thrust her hand through a glass panel'. Winifred's actions caused several superficial lacerations to her hand and arm, which were then dressed with a bandage and lint soaked in cold water to stop the bleeding. An injection of chloral hydrate was also administered.

Constant State of Excitement

On 4th November Winifred – described as being in a 'constant state of excitement' since the previous incident – was tearing at her clothing, destroying ward fittings and attempting to strike out and spit at those around her. That day, Winifred was so excited she was placed in seclusion for 1¼ hours before being given a shower bath for ninety seconds, after which – being comparatively more composed – she was placed in the day room with the other patients. Despite some fluctuations in her behaviour, by 26th December, Winifred was able to occupy herself with 'knitting and other light work' – a period of stability that lasted into the first few months of 1877. In March of that year, Winifred again suffered a serious relapse – from 25th March, Winifred's pattern of behaviour began to repeat itself whereby she would become so excited and destructive she required a draught of chloral hydrate after which she would become quieter for a short while. A few months later, on the morning of 21st July, in the course of being given a morphia injection, a bruise was noted on the right side of Winifred's face, which was thought to have been caused the day before when Winifred knocked her head against the airing court wall. After receiving the injection Winifred remained 'comparatively quiet' for the rest of the day, although this did not prevent her from being assaulted by one of the other patients. Winifred refused to have any dinner that afternoon but later walked in from the airing court to have tea. After spending some time in the day area she went to her bedroom; nothing unusual was noticed in her general demeanour at this time and the attention of nursing and medical staff was not drawn to her in any way. That night, Winifred was seen by the Night Nurse at about 9.30pm when, from her bed, she waved her arms about and shouted at the nurse in her 'usual way'. Winifred was also noisy during the early part of the night, eventually settling down before becoming noisy again at about 4am the following morning. At 5.30am Winifred was noted to be lying with her face to the wall but her body turned around as though she was about to 'spring out of bed' and attack the Night Nurse who had just entered the bedroom to check on her. The Night Nurse jumped back startled and immediately closed the door. The Night Nurse did not notice anything unduly different about Winifred and regarded the possibility of her suddenly springing up to frighten her as typical of something Winifred might do. At about 6.45am, one of the day nurses found Winifred lying on her back with some 'greenish frothy matter' about her mouth, Winifred was so stiff the nurse sought the assistance of another nurse to carry her to the day room in order to get her dressed. The two nurses were not alarmed at having to carry Winifred to the day room as she had exhibited similar behaviour in the past when it was thought she had been suffering from 'pseudo-epileptic seizures'. During such incidents, Winifred would be unable – or unwilling – to walk from her bedroom but eventually, she would usually 'come-to'. When Winifred was brought to the day room and she still did not move or speak, medical assistance was immediately summoned. On the morning of 22nd July 1877, it was found that Winifred was dead. Some of the fluid that had issued from her mouth was composed of mucopurulent matter from the bronchial tubes; bruises were noted around her eyes and there were also some small circular bruises upon her right arm apparently caused by holding her down the day before when Winifred was being given her medicine. The apparent cause of death was given as chronic mania.

SUSANNAH HALL

Date of Admission: 14th July 1870

Background

Susannah, a 50-year-old silk winder, constantly heard people talking about her and suffered from various delusions, one of which included believing – or 'fancying' – that a man by the name of Dick came to her in the night.

Admission

Following her admission, Susannah persistently talked to herself and often laughed out very loud. Over the next six months or so, 'no improvement whatever' was noted in her mental state. During this period, Susannah, described as 'this poor woman', could become very violent and was often more excitable than when first admitted. By February 1871, she was being prescribed draughts of chloral hydrate to help calm her down. When more settled, in between her periods of excitement, Susannah was allowed out into the open air 'as much as possible'.

No Improvement

Over the next few years, Susannah could be very troublesome and regularly assaulted other patients – often sustaining injuries herself as her victims were inclined to retaliate. Susannah constantly talked incoherently to no-one in particular and often waved her arms around as if warning people to keep away – sometimes even gesticulating whilst sitting with others at the dinner table. At the beginning of 1875, and now described as 'very dull of hearing' and 'quite silly looking', Susannah was nevertheless generally much quieter in her behaviour and was able to start employment as a ward helper. By August 1875, however, Susannah had started to become increasingly untidy in her appearance, had refused to work, and reverted back to making eccentric gestures and loud exclamations when conversing with others. Despite this, Susannah otherwise appeared cheerful and happy and was often fond of walking along the side of the female airing court – the side nearest the male airing court, thereby exciting the men present there 'by her manner'. Over the next eighteen months or so, Susannah remained untidy and dirty in her habits and could be very noisy at various times of the day or night but in spite of such disruptive behaviour, she presented no threat and was regarded as harmless by staff.

By March 1877, Susannah was attending Divine Service and enjoyed attending the weekly dance, even returning to her former employment as a ward helper. She could, however, still become very noisy especially when 'thwarted' by other patients or when any of them received a new dress and she didn't. A few weeks later, Susannah suffered from bursitis over the patella of her left knee; an incision was subsequently made into the wound which allowed some dark-coloured pus to be released. A linseed meal poultice was applied to the knee and Susannah was confined to bed from where she made a quick recovery. No improvement was noted in her mental state, however, and on 24th January 1878, Susannah was removed to the Third County Asylum of Middlesex at Banstead and discharged as 'not improved'.

MARGARET LAIDLAW

Date of Admission: 14th March 1877

Background

Margaret was a 33-year-old unmarried domestic servant whose address was given as 'The Infirmary, Newcastle' and who had previously been under the care of the County Asylum in Morpeth, Northumberland. According to the Senior House Surgeon there, Margaret confided to him she had drank some liniment out of a bottle on Friday, 9th March and had also attempted to drink the contents of several other bottles. It was ascertained this had indeed been the case – although Margaret was supposed to have vomited it all up again almost immediately.

Admission

On admission, Margaret stated she had written a letter to 'a woman', said to be a fortune teller, three weeks ago and that the woman – with God's permission – had transformed her into a spirit. Margaret added she felt her 'stomach was dead' and that nothing she ate passed a certain point, placing a hand on her abdomen to show where it was situated. Over the next week, Margaret remained depressed, attributing her state of mind to the supposed neglect from a young man to whom she claimed to have once been engaged. Margaret also referred to the dead feeling she had mentioned before – it had shifted higher, she said, pointing to her oesophagus as the place where this sensation was now based. By 24th March, however, the dead feeling had 'gone away entirely' with Margaret explaining her illness had originally been caused whilst still in the Infirmary by having to take some 'stuff' given to her by the fortune teller she had previously written to.

Wicked

Over the next two weeks Margaret remained in a depressed state and wept constantly; during this time Margaret wrote another letter to the fortune teller which indicated she did not have long to live. Throughout the day of 11th April, Margaret became increasingly upset at what she felt was her own wickedness, stating she ought to have killed herself when she had the chance. Margaret believed the Devil was now going to come to punish her sometime during the night. Although unable to see him, Margaret claimed to know he was there and became so frightened she promised to be his servant and do anything he wished.

Throughout the rest of April and on into May, Margaret's condition fluctuated greatly, becoming very excitable and weepy one moment before quickly calming down again and regaining her composure. When in an 'improved state' during these settled periods, Margaret was well enough to undertake some sewing in the workroom. On other occasions, however, Margaret would become distraught, fearing she had killed her aunt and sister and that the end of her own life was near – such episodes requiring draughts of chloral hydrate to be given at night to sedate her. Despite rambling in her conversation at times, by the end of May, Margaret's condition was described as 'slightly improved' and she gradually became calmer and quieter in manner. This progress proved to be short-lived, however, as on 21st June, Margaret was placed in seclusion for seven hours after becoming very excitable – by 25th June, her excitability required her to be kept in seclusion for 'some hours' every day.

Unpredictable Behaviour

During this unsettled period, Margaret refused to eat and fiercely struggled with the nurses whenever they tried to feed her; this invariably caused her to suffer a few bruises in the process – injuries regarded as 'quite unavoidable' under the circumstances. Margaret nevertheless continued to refuse food and often made 'violent efforts' to strike out at the nurses, throwing plates etc. at them whenever they attempted to give her something to eat. Even when in seclusion, Margaret would hurl her chamber-pot through the opening of the window at the top of the door-shutter. Margaret remained quite unpredictable over the following two weeks and whenever her behaviour became too unmanageable she would spend short periods of time in seclusion; occasionally, and if sufficiently settled, Margaret would be taken out to the airing court for some fresh air. Once out in the open, however, Margaret would kick out at those around her – often endangering herself by falling over in her attempts to harm others. Even when sometimes placed in a 'polka' – a dress that restricted her arms – Margaret would still lunge out, trying to bite and kick other patients – some of whom gave as good as they got by retaliating and punching her in the face. Undeterred, Margaret persisted in her disruptive behaviour – on one occasion pushing her elbows through a glass panel and being very fortunate to only suffer some bruising. On another occasion soon after this – the morning of 10th July – Margaret managed to break another glass panel and cut the palm of her left hand and was again very fortunate the wound did not require any treatment. In a further incident later that afternoon, Margaret was in a fight with another patient and thrown to the ground – her luck held out once more and no injuries were sustained. That same evening, yet more glass was broken and in this, the third incident of the day, Margaret finally injured herself by cutting her thumb and some of the fingers of her right hand, the wounds being dressed with rags soaked in carbolic oil (1 to 30). After this latest incident, Margaret was finally 'compelled' to wear a polka dress. The polka dress was briefly taken off the next morning but, owing to the 'dangerous state of excitement' Margaret was still experiencing, it wasn't long before she was put back in it again.

Later that day and in an attempt to quell her continued disruptive behaviour, Margaret was given a strong sedative, but the only effect it had was to put her into a state of intoxication – resulting in the need for Margaret to be kept under even closer observation. Once she had sobered up, Margaret remained under observation and for the next day or so, was put into a polka dress whenever she ventured out into the airing court. It was noted at this time that most of the incidents involving Margaret to date had occurred either during, or after she had been taken outside – a view soon reinforced when, out in the airing court once more, she fell and badly injured her nose. On the evening of 12th July, Margaret refused her usual meal, asking instead for bread, cheese and some porter, all of which were given to her – with a draught of chloral hydrate mixed into the porter. Margaret slept well that night and remained much quieter than usual the next day. As a result, the decision was taken for the same regime to be implemented at bedtime for the following few nights.

On the morning of 18th July, and despite becoming very excitable and 'almost unmanageable' again, Margaret was allowed out into the airing court – this time under the charge of three nurses. Such close supervision, however, did not prevent Margaret from managing to grab at the clothes of every patient who came near her as she attempted to 'hit, bite or generally tried to fight' anyone in close proximity to her. In one particular incident, Margaret had to be separated – twice – from one patient described as 'very strong and excitable'. After trying to attack this patient a third time Margaret was finally taken back to the ward, given a 'shower bath' and removed to a single room in the dormitory. Two days after this episode, Margaret's excitability had still not diminished and she endeavoured to escape from her room, tearing at a nurse's clothing as she did so and biting the fingers of one of the medical staff. It was noted that Margaret rarely sustained any injuries arising from her volatile behaviour – due mainly, it was thought, to the promptness of nurses (despite the threat of injury to themselves) in pulling her back from other patients before they had time to 'retaliate upon her'.

Spitting

In late July, Margaret suffered an 'erysipelatous inflammation' to her nose, made worse by a collection of purulent matter forming near her left eye. Because of her excited state, Margaret had to be 'partially placed under the influence of chloroform' so that an incision could be made to allow the matter to escape. After the resultant cavity was cleansed, a small piece of lint was inserted to help it heal from the inside. A 'linseed meal' poultice was then applied and secured by means of a bandage – only for Margaret to immediately tear at it and to spit the medicine she had just taken into the faces of those around her. As a result of these actions, Margaret was placed in a padded room to prevent her from further injury – but not before being 'laced up' into a polka to prevent her removing the re-applied dressings.

By 28th July, Margaret showed some signs of improving; she was now much quieter, the erysipelas was subsiding and her nose was looking much healthier – despite not allowing any dressings to remain in place for very long. The following week, however, another inflammation was noted, this time on her left arm and from which some 'very unhealthy pus' was being discharged – again, Margaret was reluctant to allow any dressings to be applied. On 3rd August, therefore, Margaret was once more put 'slightly' under the influence of chloroform and the opening which had formed on the wound was enlarged sufficiently to allow a 'quantity of dark, unhealthy pus' to be discharged. Soon after this, when the opening on her arm was examined more closely, a 'blackened and corroded' needle was found at the bottom of the incision and was subsequently removed without any difficulty. Upon further enquiry, it was discovered Margaret had previously been 'addicted' to concealing pins and needles in her mouth whenever she could get the opportunity to do so.

Annoying Everyone

From September, there was a decided improvement in Margaret's mental state and a slight improvement noted in the wounds on her nose and arm as they continued to heal. By the end of October, however, Margaret suffered a relapse and her behaviour was again becoming increasingly unmanageable day by day. Margaret was now regarded as not only volatile and unpredictable but also thought to be in constant danger from other patients if she annoyed them or attempted to steal from them. Accordingly, Margaret slept in a single room and was sometimes placed in seclusion to prevent her from coming into close contact with others but even so, she still managed on occasions – when excited – to strike out at them whenever she had the opportunity. Margaret continued in an excitable manner throughout November, annoying everyone she encountered and generally behaving in an 'exceedingly irritating' way. Having, in one incident, been prevented by a nurse from hitting another patient, Margaret later successfully approached the same patient and began to annoy her by 'pulling her about etc'. Before the same nurse could intervene again, a short scuffle ensued in the course of which Margaret was thrown to the ground where she sustained a severe contusion to the right side of her face. Margaret was immediately examined but apart from injuries to her forehead and eyebrow, there did not appear to be any damage done. Margaret was then put to bed and attempts were made to apply a dressing to her forehead. Characteristically, Margaret persistently refused to co-operate. During December, Margaret's behaviour fluctuated and whilst some improvement was noted, she continued to undergo periods of seclusion whenever she became excited and 'very troublesome'. On 21st December, and more settled than she had been previously, Margaret improved sufficiently to be able to write a letter to her friends which, after being censored, was deemed fit to be sent to them.

Signs of Improvement

After more than nine months of almost continuously disturbed behaviour, from January 1878, Margaret steadily maintained the improvement she had been making to date. Margaret now became 'far more quiet and orderly' as well as particular about her personal appearance – improvements that were sustained throughout the year. Margaret had by now given up teasing and irritating other patients but nevertheless, she was still regarded as potentially dangerous and could become easily provoked when contradicted. By April 1879, however, there was a halt to any progress made so far, when Margaret relapsed once more and started to exhibit her previous disposition to 'dangerous tendencies'. By November, Margaret was once more showing signs of improvement in her mental state and becoming tidier in her habits – she had even taken up knitting to help keep herself occupied. This time, the improvement to her mental state was sustained and by May 1880, Margaret was constantly occupied either as a ward helper or by working in the sewing room. Despite still being 'apt to become excited' when her requests were not met immediately, Margaret continued to build on this progress over the next eighteen months or so. On 7th September 1881 and four years after being admitted, Margaret was discharged home as recovered.

MARGARET O'BRIEN

Date of Admission: 12th May 1877

Background

Margaret, a 29-year-old prostitute, had previously been under treatment in the Coxlodge Asylum around three years previously. Prior to this current admission, Margaret had been described as 'excitable and loquacious', saying that two men had garrotted her and turned up her petticoats in Grey Street whilst a policeman stood by laughing.

Admission

Margaret appeared to be suffering from delirium, coughing and spitting a good deal as she stated that she 'fancied' there were a number of men in the room with her – her behaviour, however, did not appear genuine and was thought – by 'a great measure' – to be forced. Margaret's physical health was in poor condition; her skin was very dirty, her arms and legs covered in bruises and a large discoloration was noted on her abdomen. Margaret was assigned to the Second Ward and placed in a single room; later, at bedtime, she became so excited a draught of chloral hydrate was ordered to help her sleep. Having slept well, Margaret became very excited the next morning and started attacking the nursing staff; she settled down over the following week, however, and became less troublesome – only to be described as 'quiet but sulky'. On 18th May, Margaret complained of pains in her joints and a vaginal discharge; as she was noted to be menstruating, it was not possible to examine her to establish a proper diagnosis. When examined a few days later, Margaret was found to be suffering from a soft chancre on the right labium, accompanied by what was thought to be a gonorrhoeal discharge.

Unrepentant

Over the next few weeks Margaret's physical health improved although it would take another eight weeks or so for the vaginal sore to heal and, as the pains in her bones disappeared, for the various medications prescribed to treat her to be discontinued. During this period Margaret would laughingly 'narrate her misdeeds' to other patients without being in the least ashamed of what she claimed to have done. By the end of October, Margaret had become 'very quiet and well-behaved' but remained quite unrepentant over the life she had led before admission. Margaret was able to help nurses by doing chores around the ward and was even able to do a 'little fancy work' in her sewing. By 22nd December Margaret was described as 'industrious and rational' and on 24th December 1877, she was discharged as recovered.

MARY EWING

(No relation to author)

Date of Admission: 21st January 1885

Background

Mary was a 16-year-old girl whose address was given as one of Newcastle's Union Workhouses – her parents, however, lived at High Villa Place, Newcastle. Mary was one of fourteen children although nine of her brothers and sisters had died in childhood as a result of 'convulsions due to teething'. Mary herself suffered from two forms of fits with her mother claiming one type as the 'convulsive' and the other as the 'silly' – the former as a result of a 'fright' Mary received when about eight months old. The 'silly' fits were thought to have first started about eight or nine years ago and, according to her mother, have been occurring almost five or six times a day ever since. Under the influence of these particular fits, Mary would become red or purple in the face and she would sometimes lapse into unconsciousness. Often, the fits caused Mary to become irritable and unruly in the build-up to having one followed by a tendency to 'behave stupidly' after they subsided. Her mother also stated Mary was 'much addicted' to smoking and was a heavy drinker; when under the influence of alcohol Mary could become violent and strike out at those around her. According to Mrs Campbell, the 'Warden of Imbeciles' in the workhouse, Mary was 'beyond my control', adding that Mary's susceptibility to violence meant she would often break windows and assault other inmates when in a state of excitement.

Admission

During the first week of her admission, Mary proved herself to be 'passionate and mischievous', stating she had no recollection of talking to those she had been with every day, also 'quite forgetting' the pane of glass she had broken a few days into her admission. By the end of March and having suffered several major epileptic seizures, Mary was thought to be someone with both her 'intellectual and moral powers' impaired; her general disposition was also described as 'evil, vindictive, revengeful and untruthful' – especially during the periods of excitement following a seizure. Over the following months, Mary continued to behave in an excitable manner and was now in the habit of inflicting scratches etc. upon herself as well as picking off her finger nails and skin so that she could accuse the nurses of ill-treating her. On 17th September, Mary had a succession of severe epileptic seizures which confined her to bed for a few days and although she recovered well, she complained of pains in every part of her body for some time afterwards.

Rude and Abusive Language

During the next year and a half, Mary would frequently suffer from episodes of 'epileptic maniacal excitement' and continue to complain of what were regarded as imaginary bodily ailments – even though her frequent and severe seizures meant she often bruised herself falling to the ground. Generally, Mary remained in an excitable state and 'apt to be querulous', occasionally bringing charges of maltreatment against nursing staff which were never substantiated. By April 1888, Mary's condition remained unchanged and she continued to suffer from epileptic seizures after which she would generally become irritable, often using 'rude and abusive' language against those around her. On 23rd November, Mary had a series of seizures at irregular intervals between which she would be conscious and able to answer any questions put to her. Mary was prescribed various medications in an attempt to control her seizures, but these had no effect and the seizures continued – even increasing in severity on occasions. Around 8.30pm that evening, Mary lapsed into unconsciousness and her breathing became laboured; she was given an enema and at 11.30pm a hypodermic injection of ether was administered after which her pulse became stronger. During the night, however, Mary had fifteen further seizures and as the morning arrived, she became much weaker with the seizures now occurring every few minutes. At 11.30am Mary was given an increased dose of ether by injection but her condition gradually deteriorated throughout the afternoon. At 2pm, more ether was administered and she was ordered a teaspoonful of whisky every half hour – this was to be of no avail, however, as at 3.35pm on 24th November 1888, 19-year-old Mary died, the cause attributed to epilepsy.

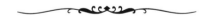

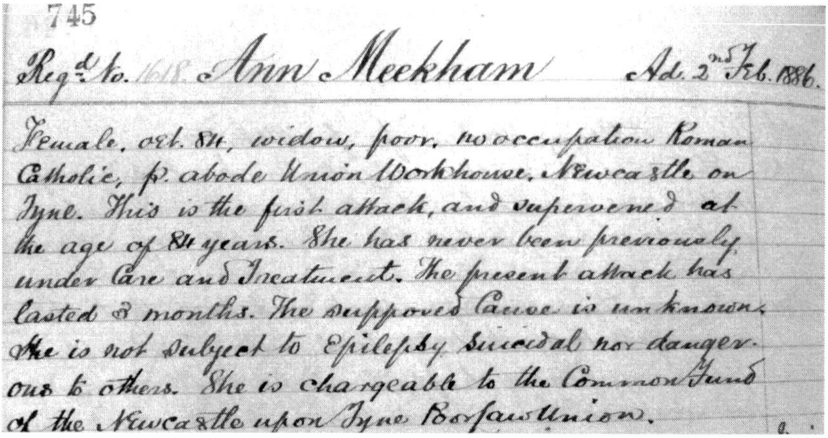

[handwritten register entry]

745

Regd to 1618 Ann Meekham   Ad. 2nd Feb. 1886.

Female, æt. 84, widow, poor, no occupation Roman
Catholic, p. abode Union Workhouse, Newcastle on
Tyne. This is the first attack, and supervened at
the age of 84 years. She has never been previously
under Care and Treatment. The present attack has
lasted 3 months. The supposed Cause is unknown.
She is not subject to Epilepsy Suicidal nor dangerous to others. She is chargeable to the Common Fund
of the Newcastle upon Tyne Poorlaw Union.

ANN MEEKHAM

Date of Admission: 2nd February 1886

Background

Ann was an 84-year-old widow whose address was given as the Union
Workhouse in Newcastle. According to Miss Campbell, Warden of Imbeciles
at the Workhouse, Ann had been wandering about at night for the last few
months in a 'restless, voluble and excited' state. As she did so, Ann would
cause a disturbance and not allow any of the other inmates to rest as she
claimed to see people around her who she imagined were out to rob her.

Admission

Ann was admitted to the Third Ward to sleep in a single room and to be visited each hour by the Night Nurse; although 'extremely voluble' and apt to
complain of imagined bodily ailments, Ann slept well that first night. Over
the following few weeks, Ann told long, loquacious stories that had 'neither
reason nor sequence' and loudly complained of imaginary injuries, pointing
to the parts of her body where they had been inflicted. Ann could become

'easily excited and exceedingly verbose' and although she generally slept well at night, she nevertheless frequently alleged someone else was in the room and would often 'beseech' staff to remove them. Throughout April and May, Ann continued to talk in the same rambling and voluble fashion, complaining of various bodily ailments and accusing men of coming into her room with the intention of 'putting an end' to her.

Frequently Complains

In the coming months, Ann was usually quite settled by day and took an interest in her surroundings – at night, however, she was apt to be noisy and sometimes inclined to sit up in bed shouting for hours at a time. As she did so, Ann would call out to her imagined people who, she says, 'come by the hundreds' to attempt to enter her room with the sole purpose of trying to kill her. Over the next few years, Ann continued in a state of 'chronic mental excitement' and she would often be very noisy, shouting and screaming at the top of her voice as she became increasingly distressed. In her agitation, Ann constantly bemoaned her fate and would say she was 'as bad as can be' and that she deserved whatever was coming to her. Despite her continued poor mental state, Ann was regarded as being in excellent general health for someone her age but by 1889 and at the age of 89, Ann was becoming physically frail. In doing so, Ann began to suffer from various ailments such as rheumatism – she remained voluble, however, and could be extremely abusive to others as a result of her delusions of persecution.

'Slight Apoplectic Seizure'

On 24th January 1890, Ann slipped on the floor of the day room and fell, injuring her right wrist; whilst no fracture could be detected, it appeared swollen and very painful to the touch. Although her arm was subsequently put in splints, Ann continually attempted to remove them with the result her arm had to be set in plaster – but she somehow managed to tear this off too. Nevertheless, Ann's wrist slowly healed and by April, she was able to move her arm freely with only a slight thickening noticeable around the wrist joint – but mentally, Ann remained very excited – and extremely noisy – both day and night. At the end of April 1891, Ann had a 'slight apoplectic seizure' and so was confined to bed for several days during which time she took very little nourishment. Not long afterwards, Ann had a similar seizure, this time accompanied by symptoms of 'pneumonic congestion' but managed to show some improvement over the next few weeks. By the end of May, Ann had returned to good general health – and also back to being 'noisy, excited and troublesome'. Throughout 1892, however, Ann's physical health declined again and by the end of the year, appeared to deteriorate further – only for her to rally round and become as noisy and troublesome as ever.

Accidentally Fell

At around midday on 29th January 1893, Ann accidentally fell while walking across the ward; on being assisted to rise she was unable to bear weight and unable to walk. As she was put to bed Ann became very excited and noisy, complaining of pain over her left hip but it was impossible to examine her properly owing to the struggle she put up. The following morning, it was noted her hip had become quite swollen and it was thought that Ann had therefore probably suffered a fractured neck of femur. Ann remained in bed with her leg kept in position by pillows; as she did not have much of an appetite, Ann was ordered a milk diet and 4ozs of whisky daily which she gradually accepted over the next few days. By the 8th February, Ann's appetite had improved although her pulse remained weak and her breathing continued to be laboured. It appeared Ann had made some kind of recovery from the shock of her fall – judging by her ever-increasing inclination to be noisy. By 14th February, however, Ann's condition had declined further – but still she managed to resist every attempt to be physically examined. By 21st February, Ann was continuing to be resistive in allowing herself to be examined although it was noted her breathing sounded as if her lungs were congested. The following morning, Ann was found to be almost unconscious; by evening she was breathing with difficulty and now 'evidently moribund'. At 11.30pm on 22nd February 1893, 93-year-old Ann died as a result of congestion and inflammation of the lungs following a fractured thigh, sustained after her recent fall.

ELIZABETH TRACEY

Date of Admission: 6ᵗʰ May 1886

Background

Elizabeth was a 25-year-old housewife who lived with her husband, Edward, in Ord Street, Newcastle. They had known each other for seven years and had been married for five of them. Elizabeth and Edward had had three children although none of them survived; Elizabeth had also suffered a miscarriage the previous year but had since given birth to a new baby only nine weeks previously. Elizabeth had grown suspicious of her husband over the last six days, hinting that he was being 'improperly intimate' with his cousin who was currently staying with them. Thereafter, Elizabeth became increasingly excitable, frequently screaming and alleging they both wished to starve her. Edward then raised concerns about Elizabeth's behaviour to the authorities and as a result, the baby – with some difficulty – was taken away from her. At the time of parting, Elizabeth was shouting to have her baby back but then suddenly seemed to forget about the baby altogether and began to 'wander in her mind and talk nonsense'. Elizabeth then alternated between episodes of laughing and crying for no apparent reason and began talking incoherently, repeating phrases such as 'those that put it in my head must take it out again'; 'what you see with your own eyes, you must believe'. Four days prior to admission, Elizabeth had gone out with a baby's frock wrapped around a poker and carried it like a baby, weeping for a priest to come and save her; the day before admission she had lain on the floor, naked, under two chairs. During this troubled time, Elizabeth had also tried to strangle herself with her long hair and had got hold of a hot poker, asking if it would serve the same purpose as a knife.

Admission

On admission, Elizabeth seemed to be of a nervous disposition and moved about uneasily as she was being physically examined; her powers of concentration were very limited and she returned irrelevant answers to the ordinary questions put to her. Elizabeth could not explain why she had been admitted nor could she give her own name upon being assigned to the Second Ward to sleep in the Infirmary Dormitory. Although Elizabeth slept well the first night, she refused to eat the following day, giving absurd answers when questioned and unable to say how many children she had or how many had survived. Over the following week, Elizabeth required feeding at mealtimes and would frequently weep without any apparent cause. By the end of the month, however, a slight improvement was noted in her mental state as she correctly replied to questions and voluntarily accepted the occasional meal.

Cheerful Disposition

It was felt Elizabeth was 'labouring under mania' and had been in a state of great mental agitation and confusion, but evidence of further improvement was now highlighted when Elizabeth began to present with a more cheerful disposition. Such progress was not sustained, however, as by 10th June, Elizabeth had suffered a relapse and was once more unable to converse intelligently. This fluctuation in Elizabeth's condition continued throughout July and August. At times, she talked rationally in a quiet and orderly manner, whilst at others, she became excited or wept like a child for no apparent reason. A slight improvement in her mental state was again noted by the end of September, progress that was maintained throughout the first few weeks of October and on 27th October 1886, Elizabeth was discharged home as 'Relieved'.

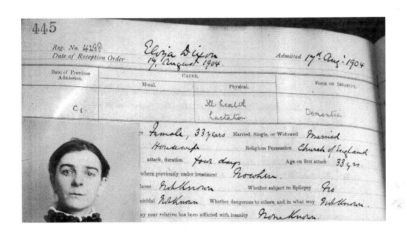

ELIZA DIXON

Date of Admission: 17th August 1904

Background

Elizabeth was a 33-year-old married housewife who lived with her husband, George, in Elswick, Newcastle. She had never been under treatment before but for the previous four days she had presented with what was described as a 'wild aspect' to her behaviour. During this period, Elizabeth wore a 'staring and vacant' expression and began talking in a rambling, irrational way – 'just a little water on the brain, I only want peace and happiness etc.' According to George, Elizabeth had become 'increasingly weak' over the past few days, thinking people had been plotting against her ever since giving birth three months previously.

Admission

On admission, Elizabeth was described as 'a small woman of sallow complexion and sharp features with a rather prominent nose, dark brown hair and dark grey eyes'; she rambled in her conversation, stating there were vermin in her hair and she appeared badly nourished. Over the next few days Elizabeth's appetite improved although her mental state fluctuated – at times she could be 'depressed, fretful and crying' whilst at others she could become 'somewhat excitable'. By the end of August, Elizabeth was a little brighter in mood and more coherent in her conversation. Whilst there was no major change noted in her mental state – Elizabeth claimed to have no idea where she was – she was showing some improvement in her general physical health. This improvement continued over the next few weeks and, as she started showing signs of improvement in her mental health, Elizabeth began to take more of an interest in her surroundings. Although not yet able to recall any memory of recent events, by the end of September, Elizabeth – now bright in mood – was occupying herself effectively in the sewing room. Elizabeth continued to make good progress throughout October and on the 19th November she was granted one month's leave on trial. Just over four months after her admission, Elizabeth was discharged home as recovered on 21st December 1904.

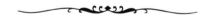

ELIZABETH MILBURN

Date of Admission: 9th June 1896

Background

39-year-old Elizabeth lived with her husband, Jeffery, at King Street, Newcastle and had been behaving strangely for the nine months prior to her admission. During that time, Elizabeth became increasingly jealous of her husband – described as an 'aged man' – and accused him of infidelity whenever he was out 'beyond his usual time'. Her behaviour towards him had become so violent that sometimes the police had to be summoned, thereby bringing them to the attention of Elizabeth's 'deluded state'. According to Jeffery, his wife had 'upbraided and quarrelled' with him many times on account of his alleged misconduct with other women, accusing him of only going out of the house to have sexual intercourse with them; according to Elizabeth, this could be with as many as twenty women in a single day. Even when Jeffery undertook an everyday activity such as going out to post a letter, Elizabeth would confront him on his return and accuse him of infidelity, often tearing at his clothes and sometimes pulling his trousers open. At other times she would get very agitated and throw things about the house, breaking dishes, plates and furniture etc.

Admission

Elizabeth was described as a 'pale, thin anaemic woman' in poor physical health with a 'sharp, excited expression' who noisily made long, rambling statements about her husband's unfaithfulness. Elizabeth eventually settled down over the next two days and was even able to take some exercise in the airing court outside. On the third day, however, she became excitable and voluble as she once more expressed 'exaggerated delusions' about her husband's alleged misconduct. Elizabeth became quieter and more restful the following week, but her delusions were still evident – nevertheless, by the end of the month Elizabeth was eating and sleeping well and an improvement in her general physical health was noted.

Not Wholly Satisfied

Throughout July as her condition improved, Elizabeth worked 'industriously' in the sewing room and appeared quiet, pleasant and tidy in her manner. She was now civil towards her husband when he visited despite there being still 'some remnant of the old delusion' left, although by the end of August, this too seemed to have disappeared altogether. As Elizabeth made further progress, she was given leave of absence from 19th September until 21st October. On her return, the asylum authorities were not wholly satisfied that Elizabeth had fully recovered and her leave was extended until the 18th November to see how she managed. Having returned on 17th November (a day early) the asylum authorities – now satisfied of her recovery – discharged her as relieved on 18th November 1896.

JANE DALGLISH

Date of Admission: 14th May 1897

Background

Jane, a 48-year-old widow suffering from 'chronic mania', had been boarded out at Sunderland Borough Asylum prior to returning to the City of Newcastle Asylum; previously, she had been under treatment at the Union Workhouse, Newcastle. Jane had become depressed and despondent, imagining that people were whispering about her and she was afraid she would do harm to someone because of the way she was feeling. Jane had become increasingly 'demented, childish and indifferent' to her surroundings with the supposed cause of her condition attributed to 'drink'.

Admission

On her admission from Sunderland Asylum, Jane looked pale and anaemic but nevertheless appeared fairly nourished; she had previously been diagnosed as having a 'soft, blowing mitral murmur' and was noted to be suffering from a patch of psoriasis on her back but otherwise, her general health was thought to be good. Mentally, Jane was deemed to be 'demented' in nature and suffering from a defective memory; she was also inclined to display occasional periods of excitable behaviour. Over the next few months, Jane laboured under chronic mania with periods of restless excitement that caused her to behave somewhat childishly. Jane, however, remained in good bodily health despite still being troubled by psoriasis although some improvement was noted by November as her 'skin eruptions' had now almost disappeared. This improvement continued into the beginning of 1898 and by the end of February her psoriasis had disappeared completely; mentally, however, Jane's behaviour remained variable as whilst she could behave childishly, she nevertheless could also be neat, pleasant and able to do her work competently on the ward.

Singing Sounds

Jane remained in a demented state with occasional attacks of restlessness or excitement, but by May she was appearing 'morbidly content' with her current circumstances. During this period Jane complained of poor hearing and continuous singing sounds in her ears. Although she could hear words in a conversation with someone who stood about a foot away from her. Jane also claimed she was unable to hear any 'whispered language' at all by those who stood beside her. By August, and over the following few months, the singing in Jane's ears gradually disappeared completely and she didn't seem quite so deaf – although any improvement in her hearing was thought to be variable. Throughout 1899, Jane remained generally 'quiet, contented and obedient'; however, she was also inclined to be dull and listless at times when she would take little interest in her surroundings – whilst continuing to be liable to the occasional outburst of excitement. Jane remained in good physical health but in February 1900 she was confined to bed for two weeks suffering from an attack of influenza. Having recovered, Jane's behaviour remained variable – she could become excitable and very emotional as she rambled in conversation but at other times, she was pleasant to talk to and easy to get on with. Over the next few years, Jane would often alternate between a state of excited restlessness and childish behaviour, to one of depression and listlessness – however, 'as a rule', Jane usually remained placid and indifferent to her circumstances.

Simple and Childish

By the end of 1905, Jane had been transferred to the Farm Ward; deemed to be in fairly good physical condition and regarded as not only simple and childish in manner but also 'petty and querulous' in behaviour. Over the next two years Jane continued unchanged and remained generally 'content with her lot', working quite happily in the sewing room. Jane still had a good appetite although her physical health fluctuated and she would frequently complain of 'small ills'. Regarded as 'simple and of feeble intellect', on 27th July, 1908, Jane – now on Ward 6 – was put to bed after having felt unwell for four days with an apparent 'syncopal attack' that left her feeling distressed. Two days later Jane had another syncopal attack followed by severe stomach pains which seemed to indicate a gradual deterioration in her physical health. On the evening of 5th August and now very frail, Jane lapsed into unconsciousness and was thought to be 'rapidly sinking'. Despite rallying the following day, Jane never quite recovered. On 8th August 1908, Jane's condition worsened and she died at 10.20 in the morning, apparently of her long-standing heart condition.

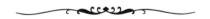

ISABELLA BOLTON

Date of Admission: 25th May 1897

Background

Isabella was a 71-year-old widow from Spital Tongues, Newcastle, whose mind, according to her son, had been 'affected' for about the past year. She had steadily been deteriorating over the past few months and was now starting to wander aimlessly around the house all day and night, getting very little rest or sleep. Isabella was becoming increasingly dependent on others to feed her at mealtimes and to help her get dressed and undressed. Isabella was initially sent to the workhouse and was only there for about a week before being transferred to the asylum; when asked how long she had been in the workhouse, she replied 'for many years' – it was felt 'no cause but old age' could be attributed to her present mental state.

Admission

On admission, Isabella was described as a 'decrepit and feeble old woman' with brown hair turning grey, grey eyes and an 'eruption of acne' on her nose and cheeks. She wore a 'vacant, stupid expression' on her face and appeared very confused, slurring in her speech as she attempted to articulate a reply in response to any questions put to her. Isabella initially found it difficult to settle but over the next few days, matters improved as she became stronger and less restless. Isabella was now more lucid and able to 'converse pleasantly' but it became increasingly evident her memory was quite impaired as she believed herself to be only 40-years-old and had been in the asylum for many months.

Feeble

On the morning of 31st May – a week after her admission – Isabella suffered a 'slight apoplexy' which left her semi-comatose and although she was soon roused from this it left her restless and unable to sleep properly. By 2nd June Isabella's condition had improved slightly, but on the 9th June it suddenly declined again and she became much weaker than before. Isabella appeared dazed and started muttering constantly to herself, managing only to accept the teaspoonful of brandy that had been prescribed for her every hour. The following day, Isabella became increasingly feeble and she was scarcely able to swallow the small amount of brandy offered to her; her skin was 'dusky and congested' and she had slept badly the previous night. Isabella remained in a semi-comatose condition throughout the 11th June before dying of 'cerebral disease' at 5am on the morning of 12th June 1897, less than three weeks after her admission.

LOUISA MONKHOUSE VASEY

Date of Admission: 27th November 1897

Background

51-year-old Louisa had been married for 20 years to her husband, Henry, an iron merchant. They lived at Hawthorn Terrace in Newcastle and had seven children, all living and healthy – the youngest, also called Henry, was only eight. According to her husband, Louisa had always been 'queer and liable to attacks of despondency' ever since the birth of little Henry. For about a week prior to her admission, Louisa had been crying constantly, fretting she had been neglecting her family and wasting money through mismanaging everything. As Louisa became increasingly restless and excited, matters took a more serious turn on the morning of Monday 22nd November when she stood by her bedside and waved a blunt carving knife across her throat. Two days later, Louisa seized a pair of scissors and attempted to cut herself, but her husband and 17-year-old son managed to wrest the scissors from her grip. Very soon after this incident, Louisa threatened to 'throttle' her children, adding that she would first take their lives before taking her own.

Admission

Louisa wore a dull and listless expression when first admitted and complained of being unable to keep her thoughts clear but despite feeling 'confused and stupid' she seemed anxious to relate all her troubles to someone. Louisa soon settled and although she slept well at night, she was nevertheless inclined to be 'depressed, morbid and emotional' in her general outlook during the day. On 30th November, Louisa was observed muttering to herself a great deal but 'stoutly denied' she was hearing voices.

Leave of Absence

Despite her denials of experiencing hallucinations and a tendency to be 'morbid and hysterical' at times, Louisa was transferred over the Christmas period to the Farm Ward where she was able to do a little sewing and help out with the housework. By the end of January 1898, Louisa's general health was improving and she appeared much brighter in mood and less pre-occupied with her 'morbid and fanciful' thoughts. This improvement was sustained over the following two weeks or so and on 16th February, Louisa was allowed to go home on leave of absence for a period of one month. However, shortly after returning home to her family Louisa became very apprehensive and was unable to sleep as she feared some sort of 'impending calamity'. As a result, Louisa was brought back to the asylum earlier than planned by her husband on 22nd February whereupon she was sent to Number 3 Ward to be kept under observation. A few days later, Louisa was transferred back to the Farm Ward where she made a quick recovery; by 17th March, Louisa was being described as 'cheerful, bright and happy' – an improvement that continued throughout April and into May. Now anxious for her to be home once more, Louisa's family and friends approached the Asylum Committee on 19th May requesting she be allowed home on leave again. Louisa's husband was accordingly permitted to take her home for another month's trial leave and on 15th June 1898, Louisa was discharged as recovered.

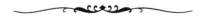

MARY YOUNG

Date of Admission: 17th March 1900

Background

Mary was a 48-year-old married woman who made a living taking in lodgers to the family home; she had also recently separated from her husband because of his 'ill treatment and drunken habits'. According to Mary's nephew, her husband was bound over to keep the peace the previous month for assaulting her, and Mary was afraid he would return to do the same again. Mary's niece added that her aunt had twice attempted suicide before; once by drinking from a bottle of laudanum – which her niece managed to take away from her – and again by attempting to throw herself from an upstairs window in her home. Mary had become very unhappy, stating she was tired of life owing to the way her husband had been treating her, adding 'he has thumped me two or three times and he is also jealous of the lodgers'. Mary thought she would never get better, saying to her niece the night before her admission that 'something could happen' – a comment which greatly concerned the niece because of Mary's previous attempts at harming herself.

Admission

Mary appeared 'dejected and dishevelled' when admitted but apart from a history of heart disease, she was in fair physical health. When interviewed, Mary plucked at her apron and tugged her ears as she complained of being tired of life, claimed to hear voices and imagined that people were pursuing her. Mary appeared depressed and found it difficult to settle during the first few days and would cry for no apparent reason – such behaviour was interspersed, however, with periods of excitement during which Mary noisily expressed delusions of persecution as she heard voices that threatened her with punishment.

Cause of Great Trouble

Over the next few months and although in fair bodily health, Mary seldom spoke and appeared depressed and listless with little interest shown in anything that was happening around her. By September, and although quiet and 'self-absorbed', Mary offered no trouble and was regarded as a fair worker in the jobs she eventually undertook around the ward. At 8pm on 5th November, and whilst the Medical Superintendent and one of the doctors were passing through the ward, Mary 'dramatically' threw herself on the floor, loosened her dress at the neck and asked that her head be cut off. At the time of the incident, Mary said she had been the cause of great trouble and should be dead – but a few days later and with a 'wild look in her eyes', claimed she didn't know what she had meant by her comments.

Mary remained depressed and emotional throughout 1901; she continued to suffer from auditory hallucinations and delusions of persecution during this period and was insistent she was living in one of 'Barnardo's Homes'. Mary remained in fairly good general physical health during this period and even though she suffered from heart disease – at present 'quiescent' – Mary was regarded as a good worker as she helped out around the ward. In March 1902, it was noted Mary was now starting to exhibit signs of mania as – in addition to her delusions of persecution – she became increasingly aggressive in her behaviour and quick to take offence. Mary's physical health and mental state remained unchanged over the next few years; at times she could be quiet and hardworking – but when excited, Mary's usual conduct was generally noisy, aggressive and threatening.

By March 1905, Mary still rambled in conversation and continued to express delusions of personal identity and persecution with such behaviour remaining quite 'unchanged in every way' over the next two years. Having previously been on Ward 5, by March 1907, Mary had been transferred to Ward 7 in an 'excited and abusive state', hearing voices and claiming to have been drugged with chloroform. A few months later, on the morning of 21st September, Mary was discovered semi-conscious by a nurse who had been called by another patient who had noticed that Mary appeared unwell. Upon examination Mary was found to be partially paralysed down the left side of her body; her right eye was shut whilst the left remained open. Mary soon lapsed into unconsciousness and at 5.15pm that evening, died from a cardiac embolism.

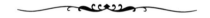

Reg. No. 3988. Date of Reception Order		Jeannie Walker. Jan 27ᵗ 1903.		Admitted Jan 27ᵗ 1903.
Date of Previous Admission.	CAUSE.			FORM OF INSANITY.
	Moral.	Physical.		
C T		Attempted forcible Seduction ?		Mania

Female, 24.
Domestic Servant.

Married, Single, or Widowed Single.
Religious Persuasion Primitive Methodist.

attack, duration about 2 weeks.

Age on first attack 24.

...here previously under treatment Never.

...use Not known.

Whether subject to Epilepsy No

...cidal No

Whether dangerous to others, and in what way No

...y near relative has been afflicted with insanity Not known

JEANNIE WALKER

Date of Admission: 27ᵗʰ January 1903

Background

Jeannie was a 24-year-old unmarried domestic servant from Pitt Street, Newcastle. This was her first episode with the apparent cause described as an 'attempted forcible seduction' that took the form of mania. According to her sister, Jeannie had been acting strangely for the past two weeks after having some trouble with a man who, she claimed, had attempted to seduce her. Jeannie had also been talking a lot of nonsense, saying such things as 'the alarm from the gasworks' did this to her and that she had also been 'nailed to the cross'.

Admission

Jeannie was not aware of where she had come from on the morning of her admission or even the day of the week. She was aggressive in manner and talked in a rambling, disconnected way. Jeannie quickly settled over the next few days and slept well at night but remained restless and resistive when awake; gradually, she became quieter and 'more sensible' over the following week. Soon, however, Jeannie became quite excitable in her general behaviour and started to assume 'strange and foolish attitudes' as she stood about the ward, gesticulating and posturing in various positions. Shortly after doing so, Jeannie reverted once more into a 'dull and stupid state' which, over the next few months, showed no signs of diminishing as she became increasingly quarrelsome and hysterical. Jeannie's behaviour started to improve again in June – but when left to her own devices she was still inclined to be aggressive if 'interfered with too much'. By November, this improvement had been sustained and whilst refusing to speak to anyone, Jeannie was nevertheless agreeable to helping out in doing a little work around the ward.

A Little Brighter

In January 1904, Jeannie was deemed to be suffering from 'mania with partial dementia' and she was once more inclined to exhibit excitable, resistive and aggressive behaviour. By April, and although still regarded as being 'dull and stupid with periods of excitement', Jeannie's mood slowly started to brighten. Jeannie maintained this gradual improvement throughout the rest of that year and well into the beginning of 1905. By July, Jeannie was demonstrating a more 'quiet, well-behaved and industrious' demeanour. On 20th September, Jeannie was given a month's leave on trial at the request of her relatives and on 18th October 1905, Jeannie was discharged as recovered.

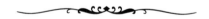

JANE SCOTT

Date of Admission: 7ᵗʰ November 1903

Background

Jane was a 33-year-old married woman of Ingham Place, Newcastle who had been experiencing some 'domestic trouble' which had resulted in an attack of mania. Jane appeared 'wild and excited' and talked in a rapid, nonsensical manner, behaving childishly and, at times, aggressively.

Admission

Jane was initially very restless and noisy when admitted but over the following few days she became a little quieter – with a tendency to be 'very silly and childish' at times. By the end of her first week, Jane would ramble in conversation and behave in a 'flighty' manner with her general conduct described as being quite 'objectionable'. The following month, however, Jane's behaviour settled down and by the end of December, her mental state had greatly improved. In January 1904, Jane's behaviour once more deteriorated as she became silly and flighty in manner and occasionally 'immodest', behaviour that remained quite unchanged over the next few months. By May, Jane had settled down again and – despite fluctuations in her behaviour – was now working well as she helped out on the ward. When unsettled, Jane continued to be restless and excitable, behave in a flighty and childish manner and was generally regarded as a nuisance to those around her. Despite this, Jane was granted a month's leave in November on the application of her relatives and, on 21st December 1904, she was discharged as relieved.

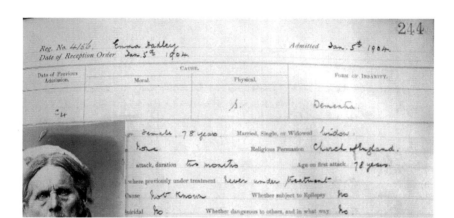

EMMA HADLEY

Date of Admission: 5th January 1904

Background

Emma, a 78-year-old widow, lived with her son, Robert, at Nary Street, Newcastle. Because of her erratic behaviour at home – described as 'very variable' – Emma had been living at the union workhouse for the past two months. Whilst at the workhouse Emma kept quietly to herself for short periods at a time – often, however, she would become restless and either attempt to tear the clothes off other inmates or strike out at them. Emma suffered from loss of memory for recent events and when asked where she was, would exclaim 'I don't know – oh yes, I'm at Newmarket. I was at home last night'.

Admission

Emma was initially restless and excitable on admission, but despite sometimes breaking down in tears, her mood nevertheless soon brightened up again. It subsequently became increasingly apparent Emma had little idea of time or place and she was thought to be suffering from senile dementia; a few days after her admission Emma thought she had been in the asylum for seven years. Over the next few months Emma's physical health improved slightly but she remained in a frail condition although this did not prevent her from behaving childishly at times. By August, Emma would either sink into periods of depression or suffer from episodes of restless excitement; her poor memory also meant she became easily confused and disorientated. Emma was now unable to tell how old she was or how long she had been in the asylum, stating she was only 23-years-old and had only been a patient for two weeks. On 31st December, Emma appeared 'very stupid, dazed and unsteady' and was sent to bed with a head cold where she soon made a quick recovery; around six weeks later, on 13th February 1905, Emma became very shaky and unsteady and so was sent back to bed again. Emma's health improved a few weeks later, having recovered from what turned out to be a sore throat and enlarged tonsils.

Pushed Over

On 15th April Emma went to the lavatory where she was pushed over by another patient, sustaining a small haematoma on the left side of the head after banging it against the wall as she fell. Emma was able to get up by herself and walk away but later complained of pain in her right hip. Whilst appearing 'much collapsed' in her general demeanour, no apparent injury was found when she was examined. The following morning Emma seemed much better – but not before badly scraping the back of her right hand after accidentally knocking it against the bedstead. Four days later, the abrasion on her hand became infected and Emma was discovered to have developed cellulitis – not only on her hand but also on her forearm where a suppurating, necrotic patch had quickly formed. The infection was treated with 'boric fomentations' but over the following two days Emma's hand and arm started to become 'oedematous and brawny' as the wound continued to discharge pus. By now, Emma was taking very little nourishment and as she became weaker her condition deteriorated further; by the evening of 22nd April Emma appeared to be sinking fast. Emma died at 9am, on the morning of 23rd April 1905 from 'heart disease; arterial degeneration and cellulitis of right hand and forearm (3 days)'.

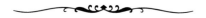

ELIZABETH JANE KIRKUP

Date of Admission: 9th January 1904

Background

Elizabeth was a 27-year-old domestic servant from Elswick, Newcastle who, for the last four weeks, had been behaving strangely – sometimes her manner was 'light and frivolous' and at other times nervous and hysterical. Although Elizabeth was apt to become excited, she often just sat on a chair chewing on her apron and pulling at it – stating on one occasion she intended to 'kill somebody'. According to her mother, Elizabeth had been complaining of violent pains in her head during this time and tended to mutter a lot as she talked to herself.

Admission

Elizabeth was admitted in a restless, excitable state, giggling and rambling incoherently whenever attempts were made to converse with her. Elizabeth quickly settled in, however, although her behaviour remained changeable as she alternated between quiet, tearful episodes and occasions when she could be 'restless and silly'. Over the next few weeks – in between quiet periods – Elizabeth was generally excitable and argumentative, often not making much sense as her conversation tended to ramble. By the end of February, Elizabeth was still generally restless and excitable and was considered 'disagreeable' by those around her because of her suspiciousness towards them – behaviour that continued over the next few months and which remained largely unchanged until the end of the year. By February 1905, however, a marked and sustained improvement was noted in Elizabeth's behaviour and she was no longer 'silly, flighty and restless'. On 15th March Elizabeth was given a month's leave on trial and on 19th April 1905, she was discharged as recovered.

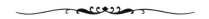

GEORGINA MATHEWS

Date of Admission: 16th April 1904

Background

Georgina, a 29-year-old unmarried woman, worked as a dressmaker and lived with her parents in Heaton, Newcastle. According to her mother, Margaret, for the previous two weeks Georgina had become depressed as she lost her appetite and started to hear voices at night. The supposed cause of her condition was attributed to shock as well as 'want of work and home trouble'. Georgina was not thought to be a danger to others although she was regarded as being suicidal and at risk of doing harm to herself.

Admission

Georgina presented as a poorly-nourished woman of 6st 2lbs with brown hair and brown eyes. Her face was described as 'very thin and pale' with a 'startled expression' as if she had 'seen or heard terrible things'. Georgina appeared to hear voices and was very frightened, crouching and shuddering as she clutched at an attendant, exclaiming with a tearful expression 'don't leave me, stay, stay!'.

A Little Brighter

During the first week Georgina found it difficult to settle and was often restless, noisy and excited; at night it was necessary to give her a draught of chloral hydrate to help her sleep. By the end of April, Georgina had improved a little, although she still heard voices – especially at night – and had to be spoon-fed as she was taking very little food.

Georgina improved both physically and mentally during May, her appetite also improved as she started to feed herself. Georgina now seemed brighter in mood and would even converse. On the occasions she was depressed, however, Georgina could become obstinate and resistive and would then refuse to speak to anyone. Over the next few months Georgina's physical health continued to improve but she remained unchanged mentally and still heard voices, her behaviour being described as generally 'dull, listless and resistive'. Some signs of improvement in Georgina's mental state were reported in October and by the following month she was noted to be 'considerably brighter' and able to converse with others quite rationally. This improvement continued throughout December to the extent that, on 18th January 1905, Georgina was granted a month's home leave on trial. Georgina was subsequently discharged recovered on 15th February 1905, weighing 6st 11lbs.

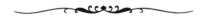

ALICE HOWITT

Date of Admission: 27ᵗʰ May 1904

Background

Alice was a 30-year-old unmarried lady with blue eyes and brown hair who lived at home with her parents at Heaton Park View, Newcastle. According to her father, Robert, Alice, who had previously been treated at Morpeth Asylum, had become 'violent, destructive and unmanageable' in her behaviour. Identifying the difficulties this caused he went on to say 'her affectations and manner have quite changed; she uses foul language and gives utterances to speech and thought quite apart from her nature. She throws things about and at anybody'. Just before her admission, Alice had wandered off to Blyth, a town just north-east of Newcastle, and had fallen into the hands of the police from whom, at the time, she had managed to conceal her identity.

Admission

When first admitted Alice was deemed to be suffering from mania with her behaviour described as 'emotional, hysterical and strange, positive and contradictory'. In responding to people she imagined she saw, heard and conversed with, Alice would grimace, gesticulate and talk incessantly, making statements such as 'I saw you this morning, do you speak French? Do you speak Italian? Bon garcon, good child, presto! You vulgar old fellow! How much do you weigh? Can you spell . . .?' etc. Alice was very flighty in her manner and attitude; she had an overwhelming opinion of her own cleverness and drew on the 'necessity' of her being provided with a husband. As she roamed around the ward singing and clapping her hands Alice rambled incoherently, destructively throwing anything 'she could get hold of'. On her first night, Alice only slept for four hours and for the next few days generally remained 'untidy, flighty, abusive and coarse in her language'.

Quiet and Well-Behaved

Throughout the month of June, Alice was much quieter and was able to moderate her language. Although she continued to ramble incoherently in conversation, Alice managed to obtain some work on the ward and became 'usefully employed'. Apart from the occasional episode of 'excitable and flighty behaviour', over the next couple of months Alice continued to be 'quiet, well-behaved and industrious'. From September, however, and over the following weeks, Alice had periods when she would be rude and offensive in conversation, mischievously breaking the windows in her bedroom after which her conduct would then improve and she became quiet and well-behaved again. By the end of October, Alice's relapses were considered worse than ever; after a period of good behaviour in November she again became excited, the observation being made that such bouts of excitement seemingly appear 'only during menstruation'. On 16th December Alice had another period of restless excitement when she became 'very flighty and objectionable' – however, by Christmas Eve she was again 'quiet and pleasant to talk to'. On 10th January 1905 Alice had another relapse, although this one was thought not to be quite so bad 'as in former attacks' and from which she soon recovered. On 12th February Alice was noted to have become restless, excited and sleepless again. On 15th March – on the petition of her relatives – Alice was discharged as 'relieved'.

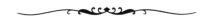

ELLEN LACKIE

Date of Admission: 3rd June 1904

Background

Ellen was a 28-year-old housewife who lived with her husband, Kenneth, in Trafalgar Street, Newcastle. Ellen had no record of previous illness but was now diagnosed with general paralysis (of the insane). For the previous two months Ellen had become vacant and listless, refusing her food and starting to behave in a strange manner. Having difficulty in finding words to express herself, Ellen tended to talk incoherently to no-one in particular as she wandered aimlessly around the house. During this time Ellen had neglected her appearance and as she became increasingly dishevelled and dirty, she would often weep and hold her head as if in pain, exclaiming she was tired of her life.

Admission

Ellen was poorly nourished and weighed only 6st 6lbs. She was described as having light brown hair and blue eyes with some large scars on both shoulders and another one at the bottom of her back. Ellen did not appear to understand the simple questions put to her but with some persuasion she managed to utter a few incoherent words in a slow and hesitating manner.

Soon after, however, Ellen began to 'talk foolishly', laughing without any apparent cause, only to then weep a great deal, crying out that she was 'sick of her rotten life' and wishing she was dead.

Unable to Understand

Throughout the rest of that month Ellen was indifferent to her surroundings and although generally quiet through the day, she tended to be restless and noisy at night which subsequently required her removal from the dormitory into a single room. Despite regaining her appetite, Ellen remained in poor physical health and exhibited 'fine tremors' of the body in association with an unsteadiness in her gait – both a consequence of the general paralysis from which she suffered. By July, Ellen's physical health improved slightly and she was being described as 'quiet but stupid', seemingly unable to understand what was said to her. Over the next few months, Ellen remained mentally unchanged but her physical health had begun to decline again; on 15th September Ellen was sent to bed owing to the 'defectiveness of the blood circulation to her extremities'. By November, Ellen was still in bed in what was described as a 'somewhat feeble condition' where she was noted to be 'dull, stupid and quite indifferent' to her circumstances. On 7th December Ellen's condition deteriorated further and she was observed to be weaker and thinner than before with her limbs 'quite useless' and 'passively placed in the one position'. By the end of December, Ellen had developed a bedsore over her sacral area with the slough coming away from the sore, leaving a 'large, raw surface' exposed. The beginning of January 1905 saw Ellen become extremely frail and taking very little nourishment – even this was taken with great difficulty as she had trouble in swallowing. All of Ellen's extremities were by now 'quite useless' and on 6th January 1905, Ellen died at 11.15pm, apparently of general paralysis.

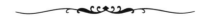

LOUISA ROBINSON

Date of Admission: 10ᵗʰ August 1904

Background

Louisa, a 'very deaf' 31-year-old woman, lived on Scarborough Road, Newcastle with her husband, William. Louisa had been married for three years and had had three children, although one of them had died of starvation; Louisa had given birth to her third child only recently. During her confinement, Louisa had been ill-treated by William – according to Louisa's mother – who used to 'knock her about'; for the last six months of her pregnancy Louisa had been 'practically starved'. Prior to her admission, Louisa had been suffering memory loss for recent events and often rambled in her conversation, saying such things as 'the curse is upon me. I heard thunder under the floor. I tell them what is going to take place beforehand. I see it in my sleep. I don't want them to do it. I hid the knife because a crime was to be committed'.

Admission

Louisa was described as a poorly-nourished woman with 'much decaying teeth', a small bruise on her left arm and the marks of recent flea bites on her legs; in addition to the heart disease she also suffered from, Louisa was now beginning to show symptoms of pulmonary phthisis. When first admitted, Louisa wore a dazed, vacant expression and rambled incoherently as she imagined that people were doing harm to her and other patients. Despite this, Louisa settled in well over the next few days although she appeared indifferent to her surroundings, remaining pre-occupied as she conducted rambling conversations in response to the voices she heard. By the end of August, Louisa showed signs of a slight improvement when she seemed to take more of an interest in her surroundings – her physical health, however, remained very poor.

Restless and Troublesome

Over the next few months, Louisa's physical health fluctuated despite an improvement in her appetite and although described as 'childish and stupid' at times, she was more often than not 'restless and troublesome' in her behaviour. During such episodes, Louisa was noisy and excitable and continually tried to find a means of escape from the ward. Her removal to a single room at night away from other patients in the dormitory was therefore necessary because of her restlessness and disruption.

By November, Louisa was exhibiting many of the symptoms of general paralysis and she showed little idea of time or place, appearing quite indifferent to her circumstances and what was happening around her. In early 1905, Louisa's physical health showed some improvement but by June it declined again as she began to suffer from the combined effects of general paralysis and pulmonary phthisis. Mentally, Louisa had no idea of time or place, stating she was 'nine million years old' and referring to herself as 'Mary, Queen of Heaven and Earth'. Despite a slight improvement to Louisa's physical health over the next few months, by November it was apparent there was a marked decline in her overall condition. Louisa was by then taking hardly any nourishment at all and she had developed a troublesome cough; at times she was incontinent of faeces with her motions noted to be 'loose, very foul and fetid'. On 24th December Louisa was described as 'extremely thin and frail'; she slept very badly and tolerated milk as her only means of nourishment. Louisa became increasingly weaker over the next few days, however, and lapsed into unconsciousness. At 4.55pm on 29th December 1905, Louisa died from pulmonary phthisis and general paralysis.

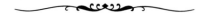

Glossary of Common (and Less Common) Terms

Abscess – A swelling in soft tissue filled with pus caused by an infection, such as a boil. *(www.thornber.net)*

Acetate of Morphia – See Morphine.

Airing Court – A yard enclosed by walls . . . 'A place where patients suffering from maniacal excitement might work off their morbid energy in safety' (. . . 'they may also be a source of irritation and annoyance to those confined in the airing court along with them'). *(www.studymore. org.uk)*

Ataxic Gait (Ataxia) – An inability to co-ordinate voluntary muscular movements – including gait – that is symptomatic of some disorders of the central nervous system. See also Chorea. *(www.merriam-webster.com)*

(The) Big House – A staff reference to the asylum as a whole. *(A History of St Nicholas Hospital, Newcastle-upon-Tyne, England 1869 – 2001)*

Belladonna Plaster – Belladonna – also known as deadly nightshade – was grown in monastery gardens during medieval times and used to treat inflammations and boils. From 1900-1930 belladonna was softened through heating and spread onto a strip of fabric or similar backing and applied where needed. People used it to relieve the pain of conditions such as lumbago, rheumatism and sciatica. *(www.rpharms.com)*

Bismuth and Pepsin Mixture – Now used to soothe upset stomachs, it was originally developed at the start of the 20th century, when standards of hygiene and sanitation were poor, to treat severe diarrhoea and vomiting – often the symptoms of diseases such as cholera. *(www.pepto-bismol.com/en-us/about/history)*

Boric (Acid) Fomentation – Fomentation: the application of a hot moist substance to the body to ease pain. *(www.merriam-webster.com)* Boric acid: Often used as a mild antiseptic, especially on yeast and fungal infections; is an effective treatment for some skin conditions such as mild rashes and acne. *(www.healthfully.com/medical-use-boric-acid)*

Bread Poultice – See Poultice.

Bromide of Potassium – Historically, thought to be of benefit in 'subduing irritation in hysteria, and in procuring sleep in nervous persons' as well as in the treatment of epilepsy. *(www.doctor-treatment.com)*

Bronchitis – Irritants, or infectious organisms enter the airways of the lungs resulting in inflammation and a mucous-producing cough; in the form of a long-standing, repetitive condition, it is called chronic bronchitis which results in protracted and often permanent damage to the lungs. *(www.britannica.com)*

Cancer – A malignant tumour of potentially unlimited growth that expands locally by invasion and systemically by metastasis. *(www.merriam-webster.com)*

Canker (Sores) – Small, painful ulcers of the oral cavity; these are round, shallow, white ulcers on the inner surface of the cheek or lip. *(www.britannica.com)*

Canvas Straitjacket – See Straitjacket.

Canvas Suit – See Straitjacket.

Camisole – A tight-fitting coat of heavy canvas with no buttons, reaching from neck to waist. The sleeves of the camisole are closed at the ends, and the jacket, having no opening in front, is adjusted and tightly laced behind. To the end of each blind sleeve is attached a strong cord, the one on the right carried to the left of the body, and the cord on the left carried to the right of the body. Both are then drawn tightly behind, thus bringing the arms of the patient into a folded position across his chest with the cords then securely tied. *(Clifford Beers, A Mind that Found Itself: An Autobiography, 1923)* See also Straitjacket.

Carbolic (Acid) Oil – A strong disinfectant which may be used for disinfecting the skin before surgery; in the proportion of one ounce to 40 ounces of water it may also be used for disinfecting 'foetid ulcers and certain purulent sores'. When diluted to one pint in 200 pints of water, it forms a gargle for sore-throats 'attended with foetid breath'. *(www.doctortreatments.com/19th-century-medicines)*

Carbuncle – A type of inflammatory infection of the skin. A carbuncle typically consists of two or more interconnected boils called furuncles; these are painful red nodules that form yellowish heads which burst to release pus and dead tissue. They occur most often in hairy skin areas or areas that are subject to friction, for example, the back of the neck, the armpits, and the buttocks. *(www.britannica.com)*

Cardiac Dyspnea (Dyspnoea) – Pertaining to the heart or to the upper part of the stomach and a shortness of breath associated with congestive heart failure. *(www.oxfordreference.com)*

Castor Oil – A thick yellowish liquid that comes from the seeds of the castor bean and is used as a lubricant and as a strong laxative. *(www.merriam-webster.com)*

In the 19th century, constipation was believed to exacerbate insanity and patients were frequently subjected to a wide variety of drastic purgatives and emetics including castor oil to alleviate its symptoms. *(Sketches From the History of Psychiatry – BJPSYCH Bulletin: pb.rcpsych.org/content/pbrcpsych/13/8/440.full.pdf)*

Catatonic (or Manic) Excitement – A definition of a type of schizophrenia: the person will be in a state of almost complete immobility, characterised by mutism or extreme compliance, preceded or interrupted by episodes of excessive motor activity and excitement; a condition whereby sufferers are generally impulsive and unpredictable. *(www.lib.uwo.ca)* See also Mania.

Chancre – **A** typical skin lesion of the primary stage of syphilis usually appearing on the penis, labia, cervix, or anorectal region. (In women, the chancre often occurs internally and therefore may go unnoticed.) *(www.britannica.com)* See also Syphilis.

Chloral Hydrate – Also called chloral, the first synthetically produced sedative-hypnotic drug commonly used in the late 19th century to treat insomnia; a therapeutic dose produces a deep sleep lasting four to eight hours with few after-effects, although habitual use of the drug can result in addiction. *(www.britannica.com)*

Colic – A sharp abdominal pain with an acute onset that can be due to contraction of the smooth muscle of the intestinal, renal or biliary tracts, or blockage with kidney stones or gallstones. *(www.oxfordreference.com)*

Colitis – Inflammation of the colon; ulcerative colitis – of unknown cause – varies from a mild inflammation of the mucosa of the rectum to a more severe, sudden illness, with destruction of a large part of the colonic mucosa, considerable blood loss, toxaemia and, less commonly, perforation. *(www.britannica.com)*

Chorea – A disorder of the central nervous system characterised by uncontrollable brief jerky movements mainly of the face and extremities. *(www.thornber.net)*

Chronic Bronchitis – See Bronchitis.

Chronic Mania – See Mania.

Coma – A state of unarousable unconsciousness. *(www.oxfordreference.com)*

Congestion – Accumulation of blood or other fluid in a body part or blood vessel, for example, congestion of the lungs in a failing heart; in congestive fever the internal organs become gorged with blood. *(www.thornber.net)*

Consumption – A wasting away of the body, formerly applied to illnesses such as pulmonary tuberculosis. In 'Physick, it is a waste of muscular flesh frequently attended by a hectick fever'. *(www.thornber.net)*

Convulsions – Involuntary contraction of the muscles producing contortion of the body and limbs. *(www.oxfordreference.com)* See also Epilepsy.

Cyanide Gauze – An antiseptic dressing where the gauze is impregnated with cyanide of mercury and zinc (as developed by Joseph Lister). *(www.kingscollections.org/antiseptic-dressings)*

Delusions – A rigid system of beliefs with which a person is preoccupied and to which the person firmly holds, despite the logical absurdity of the beliefs and a lack of supporting evidence. Delusions are symptomatic of mental disorders such as schizophrenia and major depression. Among the most common are delusions of persecution and grandeur. *(www.britannica.com)*

Delusions of Persecution – See Delusion.

Dementia – By the 18th century, dementia was described as a 'state of acquired intellectual deficit with behavioural connotations, at any age and of any cause' – a young adult with serious head injuries, for example, might be labelled as having dementia. The label was also applied to severe psychotic illnesses, which were thought of as dementing processes (leading to Kraeplin's diagnosis of 'dementia praecox', the forerunner of schizophrenia). By the end of the 19th century, a diagnosis of dementia tended to be confined to patients with a loss of cognitive ability – senile dementia as it is now understood was not described until the beginning of the 20th century. *(S.A. Hill; R. Laugharne, Journal Royal Society of Medicine, July 2003, Vol. 96, No. 7, P. 361-363)*

Depression – A mood or emotional state marked by feelings of low self-worth or guilt; it may be characterised by symptoms such as feelings of sadness, hopelessness, or pessimism as well as disturbed sleep and a loss of appetite. *(www.britannica.com)* Depression may or may not be triggered by stressful events or trauma; risk factors include genetic and social elements. *(www.oxfordreference.com)* See also Melancholia.

Discharged: After 14 Days – If patients are absent from the asylum for longer than this period they are regarded as no longer mentally ill; discharge usually occurs after a period of temporary absence such as leave. Patients who escaped would be regarded as 'temporarily absent' and subsequently discharged – if they were not 'retaken' within the 14-day period. **Recovered** – Recovery made from episode of mental illness and treatment no longer required. **Not Recovered** – Recovery incomplete but discharge granted on the application of a friend or relative as long as the patient was properly taken care of. **Relieved:** Patient not considered recovered but taken away by family – or possibly returned to the work-house. *(www.studymoreorg.uk)*

Dressing Plug – A small wad of dressing material, such as lint, used either to cover a wound or sore; it was also used during operations, mounted on an instrument, to wipe away blood or to stem its flow. *(www. oxfordreference.com)*

Dysentery – Inflammation of the intestine; symptoms include 'contagious pyrexia (fever)' and 'frequent griping stools'. It has also been described as 'a disease in which the excrements are mixed with blood'. *(www. thornber.net)*

Dyspnoea – Laboured or difficult breathing; can be due to obstruction to the flow of air into and out of the lungs as in bronchitis and asthma, or in various diseases affecting the tissue of the lung such as emphysema and tuberculosis. *(www.oxfordreference.com)*

Enema – A quantity of fluid infused into the rectum through a tube passed into the anus to remove faeces. *(www.oxfordreference.com)*

Emphysema – Air in the tissues: where the air sacs (alveoli) of the lungs are enlarged and damaged, causing breathlessness which can be made worse by infection. *(www.oxfordreference.com)*

Epilepsy – A disorder of the nervous system, characterised by mild and occasional loss of attention or sleepiness (petit mal) or by severe convulsions with loss of consciousness (grand mal); various disorders marked by abnormal electrical discharges in the brain and typically manifested by sudden brief episodes of altered or diminished consciousness, involuntary movements, or convulsions. *(www.merriam-webster.com)*

Epithelioma – *Epithelium:* the covering of internal and external surfaces of the body; a membranous tissue that serves to enclose and protect other parts of the body. *Epithelioma:* a benign or malignant tumour derived from epithelial tissue. *(www.merriam-webster.com)*

Erysipelas – Characterised by large, raised red patches on the skin (especially the face); painful, very red, swollen, and warm skin underneath sores (lesions); a type of skin infection (similar to cellulitis) with symptoms that include fever, shaking, and chills. *(www.jenwilletts.com/ 19thCenturyMedical)*

Ether A volatile liquid used as an anaesthetic administered by inhalation. *(www.oxfordreference.com)* By intravenous injection: to induce unconsciousness rapidly and avoid the unpleasantness of an inhalational induction. *(www.oxfordreference.com: Anesthesia, General. The Oxford Companion to the Body)*

Fomentations – A preparation of hot moist material applied to any part of the body to increase local circulation, alleviate pain, or soften the skin to allow matter to be expressed; cloth steeped in hot water and applied to 'a sore place' or wound such as a boil. *(www.oxfordreference.com)* See also Poultice.

General Paralysis (of the Insane) – Otherwise known as General Paresis or 'Dementia Paralytica', a neuropsychiatric disorder – caused by syphilitic infection – which affects the brain and central nervous system. *(www. studymoreorg.uk)*

A disease of the central nervous system, it is a late manifestation of syphilis often occurring up to 15 years after the original infection and characterised by mental deterioration, speech defects and progressive paralysis. *(www.collinsdictionary.com)*

See also Syphilis.

Gonorrhoea – Sexually transmitted disease characterised by inflammation of the mucous membranes of the genital tract. *(www.oxfordreference.com)*

Hallucinations – A false perception of something that is not really there; may be visual, auditory, tactile, gustatory (of taste), or olfactory (of smell). They may be provoked by mental illness such as schizophrenia or severe anxiety disorders; physical disorders affecting the brain such as temporal lobe epilepsy, sepsis, acute organic syndrome, or stroke; they may also be caused by drugs or sensory deprivation. *(www. oxfordreference.com)*

Hemiplegia (Hemiparesis) – Paralysis of one side of the body; caused by disease affecting the opposite (contralateral) hemisphere of the brain. *(www.oxfordreference.com)*

Hypertrophy of the Heart (Cardiomyopathy) – A condition affecting the heart characterised by unexplained thickening (Hypertrophy) of the wall of the left ventricle. *(www.oxfordreference.com)*

Hypochondria – A preoccupation with the physical functioning of the body and with imagined ill health; in the most severe form there are delusions of ill health, often associated with underlying illness, such as depression. *(www.oxfordreference.com)*

See also Delusion.

Hypodermic Injection (Syringe) – Surgical instrument for injecting fluids beneath the skin into a muscle or blood vessel. It comprises a graduated tube containing a piston plunger, connected to a hollow needle. *(www. oxfordreference.com)*

The injection of a medicine or drug under the skin. *(www. collinsdictionary.com)*

Imbecile – Entered English in the mid-16th century as an adjective meaning (mainly physically) weak, or impotent. Via French from the Latin for "without support". It acquired its meaning of mentally weak in the early 19th century. Congenital Imbecility is the result of some original defect, which renders the mind feeble in all its operations, though not altogether incapable of exercising them within a limited sphere. *(www. studymoreorg.uk)*

Impetigo – Inflammatory skin infection that begins as a superficial blister or pustule then ruptures to give rise to a weeping spot on which the fluid dries to form a distinct honey-coloured crust; may be spread by poor hygiene and crowding and is a particular problem in humid, hot weather. *(www.britannica.com)*

Intemperance – A lack of moderation, especially of habitual or excessive drinking of intoxicants. *(www.merriam-webster.com)*

Iron Mixture – See Tincture of Iron.

Linseed Meal Poultice – See Poultice.

Linseed, oil and Mustard Poultice – See Poultice.

Lobar Pneumonia – See Pneumonia.

Locked Gloves – Used to prevent patients from harming themselves; small padded canvas bags tied around the wrists to prevent injury or destructiveness; one description of a locked canvas glove is given as a 'pear-shaped, white, canvas mitten, stitched in black around the edges with sewn-on canvas wrist-strap and brass buckle with lock. The lock is a small torpedo-shaped, screw-in bolt which is turned with a key'. (It has been suggested that locked gloves were particularly employed to discourage masturbation – considered a possible cause of insanity until as late as 1939). *(www.collections.museumvictoria.com.au/items/249301)*

Mania – A state of mind characterised by excessive cheerfulness, grandiose delusions and increased activity; the mood is euphoric and can change rapidly to irritability. Thought and speech are pressured and rapid to the point of incoherence and connections between ideas may be difficult to follow. Behaviour is overactive, extravagant, overbearing and sometimes violent. *(www.oxfordreference.com)*

See also Catatonic Excitement.

Melancholia (The 'Melancholies') – There were thought to be several degrees and varieties; some displayed merely lowness of spirits with a distaste for the pleasures of life, and a total indifference to its concerns; they had no defect in intellectual powers and manifested no delusion or hallucination. Others derived their grief and despondency from some unreal misfortune, which they imagined to have befallen them. Many were convinced they had committed unpardonable sins or some heinous crime and were doomed to eternal perdition. A proportion of melancholy patients lived under the impression they laboured under some terrible bodily disease and magnified the symptoms of minor complaints into an 'incurable distemper', often attributed to some 'fantastical cause'. *(www.studymoreorg.uk)*

Mental Derangement – The state of being mentally ill and unable to think or act in a controlled way. *(www.collinsdictionary.com)*

Morphine – Isolated from opium; initially used to sedate patients and induce long periods of sleep, now most often used as a powerful painkiller. *(www.lib.uwo.ca)*

Muriate Tincture of Iron – See Tincture of Iron.

Parole – Conditional release of a formally committed patient; a system of supervision for patients who are allowed to leave the asylum but who may be returned at any time without the need for further court action; also called 'trial' or 'day' leave. *(www.medical-dictionary.thefreedictionary.com)*

Paroxysm – A sudden violent attack, especially a spasm or convulsion. *(www.oxfordreference.com)* See also Convulsion and Epilepsy.

Parturition – The act of giving birth. *(www.oxfordreference.com)* See also Puerperal Insanity.

Petit-mal – A specific form of epilepsy characterised by a transient, subtle impairment of consciousness. Also known as absence seizure, it denotes a period of three 30 seconds duration in which ongoing motor activities such as talking, eating, or walking cease and the sufferer stares ahead, seemingly unseeing, unhearing, and uncommunicative. *(www. oxfordreference.com)* See also Epilepsy.

Phthisis – Greek word meaning 'a dwindling or wasting away' (pronounced Tie-sis); an old name for the wasting disease Tuberculosis. *(www. medicinenet.com)* A chronic wasting away due to lung disease; also known as tuberculosis or consumption. *(www.jenwilletts.com/19thCenturyMedical)* See also Tuberculosis and Consumption.

Pneumonia – An acute, infectious disease marked by inflammation of lung tissue and characterised by fever, chills, coughs, difficulty in breathing, fatigue, chest pain and reduced lung expansion. *(www.merriam-webster. com)*

Polka Dress – See Straitjacket; Camisole.

Poultice – A soft moist mass of bread, meal, clay, or other adhesive substance usually heated, spread on cloth, and applied to warm, moisten, or stimulate an aching or inflamed part of the body. *(www.medical-dictionary. thefreedictionary.com)*

Psoriasis – A chronic disease in which scaly pink patches form on the elbows, knees, scalp, and other parts of the body; may occur in association with arthritis. *(www.oxfordreference.com)*

Puerperal Insanity (Fever) – A rare, acute mood disorder that sometimes occurs in women after childbirth, characterised by a severe manic reaction. *(www.medical-dictionary.thefreedictionary.com)* A fever arising after giving birth, also called child bed fever, caused by bacterial infection and commonly fatal until the introduction of sulphonamides and later antibiotics in the middle of the 20th century. *(www.thornber.net)* See also Mania.

Pulmonary Tuberculosis – See Tuberculosis.

Pulmonary Phthisis – See Phthisis.

Religious Exaltation – *Religious Experience:* A specific experience such as wonder at the infinity of the cosmos; a sense of awe and mystery in the presence of the sacred or holy; a feeling of dependence on a divine power or an unseen order. *(www.britannica.com) Exaltation:* A state of cheerful excitement and enthusiasm; a marked elation of mood. *(www. oxfordreference.com)*

Seclusion – The act of placing or keeping someone away from other people (for their own or other people's safety). *(www.merriam-webster.com)*

Scabies – A skin infection caused by the mite *Sarcopetes;* typified by severe and intense itching (particularly at night), red papules, and often secondary infection. *(www.oxfordreference.com)* Contagious itch or mange with exudative crusts caused by parasitic mites. *(www.merriam-webster.com)*

Senile Dementia – See Dementia.

Seizures – A disorder of the central nervous system characterised by periodic loss of consciousness with or without convulsions. In some cases it is due to brain damage but in others the cause is unknown. *(www. collinsdictionary.com)* See also Epilepsy.

Shower Bath – Water was thought to be an effective treatment because it could be heated or cooled to different temperatures, which, when applied to the skin, could produce various reactions throughout the rest of the body. Warm continuous baths were used to treat patients suffering from insomnia, those considered to be suicidal and assaultive, and calmed excited and agitated behaviour. Packs consisted of sheets dipped in varying temperatures of water, which were then wrapped around the patient for several hours depending on the case. Sprays functioned like showers, and used either warm or cold water. Cold water was used to treat patients diagnosed with psychosis and those showing signs of 'excitement and increased motor activity'. *(www.lib.uwo.ca)*

Sleeping Draught – Any drink containing a drug or agent that induces sleep. *(www.collinsdictionary.com)* See also Chloral Hydrate.

Soda Hydrosulphur (Sodium Hydroxide) Lotion – A type of soap; lye (sodium hydroxide mixed with liquid) and oil molecules chemically combine to form a soap; also referred to as lye soap. *(www.chagrinval-leysoapandsalve.com)*

Spirits of Ammonia – Hydroalcoholic solution used mainly by inhalation to produce reflex stimulation in people who have fainted or are at risk of syncope; also referred to as 'smelling salts'. *(www.medical-dictionary. thefreedictionary.com)*

Straitjacket (or Straightjacket) – A garment shaped like a jacket with over-long sleeves, typically used to restrain a person who may otherwise cause harm to themselves or others. Once the arms are inserted into the straitjacket's sleeves, they are then crossed across the chest. The ends of the sleeves are then tied to the back of the wearer, ensuring that the arms are kept close to the chest with as little movement as possible. *(www.englishdictionary.education/en/straightjacket)* See also Camisole.

Strong Rug – Controversial method of restraint used by some Medical Superintendents: locking naked patients in a side room sometimes for weeks at a time; they slept on the floor without either bed or pillow, being supplied only with strong, quilted rugs. *(www.islingtontribune. com/news/2010/oct/bedlam-shell-shock)*

Sulphur Ointment – The cleansing power of 'sulphur' has been known for centuries; ancient physicians burned sulphur in a house to cleanse it of impurities; creams made with sulphur were used to treat infections and diseases. *(www.encyclopedia.com)* A non-metallic element that is active against fungi and parasites. It is a constituent of ointments and other preparations used in the treatment of skin disorders. *(www. oxfordreference.com)*

Syncope (Syncopal Attack) – Fainting; loss of consciousness due to a sudden drop in blood pressure resulting in a temporarily insufficient flow of blood to the brain; it may also be caused by an emotional shock or by standing for prolonged periods. *(www.oxfordreference.com)*

Syphilis – A venereal disease caused by infection and characterised by an ulcerating chancre, usually on the genitals and processing through the lymphatic system to nearly all tissues of the body. *(www.collinsdictionary. com)*

Syphilitic Rash – See Syphilis.

Tincture of Iron – A combination of herbs noted for their high iron content and for their success in increasing iron levels in the blood; a herbal tonic that also relieves constipation. *(www.herblore.com)*

Tincture of Potassium Chloride – An antiseptic for use on minor wounds, cuts and abrasions. *(www.medicines.org.uk)*

Tuberculosis – An infectious inflammatory disease that is chronic in nature and especially affects the lungs, although it may spread to other areas such as the kidneys or spinal column; a serious disease that mostly affects the lungs and is associated with fever, cough and difficulty in breathing. *(www.merriam-webster.com)*

Transfer (Transferring Patients) – The act of moving a person with limited function from one location to another. *(www.medical-dictionary. thefreedictionary.com)*

References

Introduction

The Architectural Image of the Asylum by Dr Jeremy Taylor

Taken from:
Mind Over Matter – A study of the Country's Threatened Mental Asylums (Page 15)

A Report by:
SAVE Britain's Heritage, 1995 (Out of Print)

A History of St Nicholas Hospital, Newcastle upon Tyne
England 1869 – 2001 by Logan Ewing, Authorhouse, (2009)
www.authorhouse.co.uk

Male

All case histories taken from case books (Reference: HO.SN.13.1 – 51) which are stored at Tyne and Wear Archive Services, Blandford House, Newcastle upon Tyne.

Website: www.twarchives.org.uk/collection/catalogue

William Bannan:
HO.SN.13.4 Page 167

David Bell:
HO.SN.13.3 Page 171

Thomas Bruce:
HO.SN.13.3 Page 379
HO.SN.13.4 Page 72
HO.SN.13.5 Page 40
HO.SN.13.6 Page 61
HO.SN.13.9 Page 45

Max Freudenthal:
HO.SN.13.3 Page 193

Peter Gallagher:
HO.SN.13.3 Page 369

Patrick Henry:
HO.SN.13.2 Page 16
HO.SN.13.3 Page 49

William Skeldon Hodgson:
HO.SN.13.3 Page 509

Henry Scott Hood:
HO.SN.13.3 Page 829
HO.SN.13.4 Page 102

Robert Littlewood:
HO.SN.13.3 Page 367

Charles Saville:
HO.SN.13.2 Page 160
HO.SN.13.3 Page 78
HO.SN.13.4 Page 39

Thomas Henry Shaw:
HO.SN.13.2. Page 476

William James Taylor:
HO.SN.13.1 Page 80
HO.SN.13.3 Page 11
HO.SN.13.4 Page 9
HO.SN.13.5 Page 6
HO.SN.13.6 Page 46
HO.SN.13.9 Page 9

William Ainsley:
HO.SN.13.5 Page 876
HO.SN.13.6 Page 155
HO.SN.13.9 Page 141

William Best:
HO.SN.13.7 Page 403

Thomas Caverhill:
HO.SN.13.5 Page 617
HO.SN.13.6 Page 126
HO.SN.13.9 Page 111

Hugh Begg Clerk:
HO.SN.13.7 Page 417
HO.SN.13.9 Page 267

John Dick:
HO.SN.13. 4 Page 514
HO.SN.13.5 Page 63
HO.SN.13.6 Page 72
HO.SN.13.9 Page 67

John Henry Gibson:
HO.SN.13.3 Page351
HO.SN.13.4 Page 68
HO.SN.13.5 Page 38
HO.SN.13.6 Page 143

Joseph Hope:
HO.SN.13.8 Page 454
HO.SN.13.9 Page 423

William McAllister:
HO.SN.13.6 Page 477
HO.SN.13.9 Page 153

William Reed:
HO.SN.13.8 Page 160
HO.SN.13.9 Page 369

Joseph Routledge:
HO.SN.13.5 Page 359
HO.SN.13.6 Page 141
HO.SN.13.9 Page 91

James Smith:
HO.SN.13.4 Page 323
HO.SN.13.5 Page 68
HO.13.6 Page 75
HO.SN.13.9 Page 103

John Tindall:
HO.SN.13.7 Page 408
HO.SN.13.9 Page 251

Female

All case histories taken from case books (Reference: HO.SN.13.1 – 51) which are stored at Tyne and Wear Archive Services, Blandford House, Newcastle upon Tyne.

Website: www.twarchives.org.uk/collection/catalogue

Isabella Bolton:
HO.SN.13.35 Page 385

Annie Buckley-Smith:
HO.SN.13.31 Page 767
HO.SN.13.32 Page 126

Mary Ewing:
HO.SN.13.31 Page 595
HO.SN.13.32 Page 75

Susannah Hall:
HO.SN.13.2 Page 310
HO.SN.13.30 Page 98

Ann Knight:
HO.SN.13.1 Page 120
HO.SN.13.30 Page 41
HO.SN.13.31 Page 37

Margaret Laidlaw:
HO.SN.13.30 Page 577
HO.SN.13.31 Page 96

Winifred Malan:
HO.SN.13.2 Page 6
HO.SN.13.30 Page 60

Ann Meekham:
HO.SN.13.1 Page 745
HO.SN.13.32 Page 112

Elizabeth Milburn:
HO.SN.13.35 Page 181

Margaret O'Brien:
HO.SN.13.30 Page 605

Elizabeth Tracey:
HO.SN.13.31 Page 797

Louisa Monkhouse-Vasey:
HO.SN.13.35 Page372

Jane Dalglish:
HO.SN.13.35 Page 370
HO.SN.13.39 Page 47

Elizabeth Dixon:
HO.SN.13.38 Page 445

Emma Hadley:
HO.SN.13.38 Page 244

Alice Howitt:
HO.SN.13.38 Page 373

Elizabeth Jane Kirkup:
HO.SN.13.38 Page 250

Ellen Lackie:
HO.SN.13.38 Page 382

Georgina Mathews:
HO.SN.13.38 Page 328

Louisa Robinson:
HO.SN.13.38 Page 442

Jane Scott:
HO.SN.13.38 Page199

Isabella Stult:
HO.SN.13.30 Page 242
HO.SN.13.31 Page 62
HO.SN.13.32 Page 25

HO.SN.13.34 Page 49
HO.SN.13.39 Page 21

Jeannie Walker:
HO.SN.1338 Page 1

Mary Young:
HO.SN.13 36 Page 259
HO.SN.13.39 Page 39